Think Like a Nurse
A Handbook

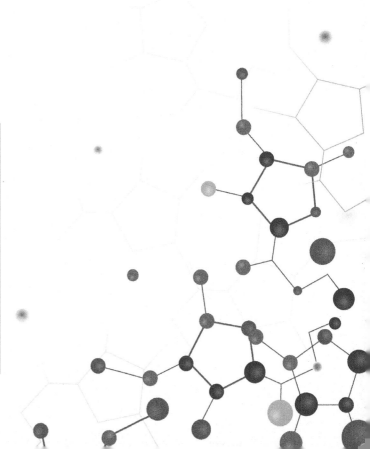

Think Like a Nurse
A Handbook

Linda Caputi,
RN, MSN, EdD, CNE, ANEF

Recommended by the
National Council of State Boards of Nursing
as a sophisticated method for teaching clinical judgment
to prepare students for the Next Generation NCLEX
www.ncsbn.org/13487.htm

WINDY CITY
PUBLISHERS

Think Like a Nurse
A Handbook

Windy City Publishers
2118 Plum Grove Road, #349
Rolling Meadows, IL 60008

www.windycitypublishers.com

Published in the United States of America

ISBN:
978-1-941478-49-3

Library of Congress Control Number:
2017947431

WINDY CITY PUBLISHERS
CHICAGO

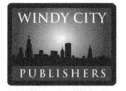

I am honored to dedicate...

this book to all nursing faculty and staff educators who, like me,
have been searching for the answer to how to teach students and nurses
to **_think like a nurse_**.

I discovered that students and nurses must first **develop** clinical judgment
before they can be asked to **use** clinical judgment.
This is the missing piece for which I searched for nearly 20 years.

Once clinical judgment is **developed**, it can then be **used**.
Once I discovered this missing piece around 1998,
I developed the _Caputi Model for Teaching Thinking in Nursing_,
implemented the model, and discovered it worked!
I continued to revise and refine that model over the next
ten to fifteen years to where the model is today.

It is my hope this book can help others so their struggle with learning
to teach thinking in nursing will not span two decades as mine did!

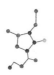

About the Author

Linda Caputi,
MSN, EdD, CNE, ANEF

Dr. Caputi is Professor Emeritus, College of DuPage, after teaching over 27 years. She has taught in LPN, ADN, BSN, and MSN programs. She has won six awards for teaching excellence from Sigma Theta Tau, is included in 3 years of *Who's Who Among America's Teachers*, and was nominated for the Outstanding Teacher Award in 2005 from the National League for Nursing. She won the Educator of the Year Award in 2004 from the National Organization for Associate Degree Nursing Foundation.

Linda Caputi is President of Linda Caputi, Inc., a nursing education consulting company. Dr. Caputi has consulted with hundreds of schools over the last 20 years on topics related to revising curriculum, preparing for accreditation, teaching students to think, developing a concept-based curriculum, transforming clinical education, writing test items and test construction, using an evidence-based model for NCLEX success, and numerous other nursing education topics. She has conducted hundreds of faculty development workshops, spoken at numerous nursing education conferences, and given many keynote addresses over the last 30 years.

Dr. Caputi co-authored *Mastering Concept-Based Teaching: A Guide for Faculty* with Drs. Giddens and Rodgers published by Elsevier. Dr. Caputi has edited four books published through the NLN in the last 4 years and has written numerous book chapters and journal articles. The 2nd edition of her book *Teaching Nursing: The Art and Science* won the 2010 Top Teaching Tools Award in the print category from the *Journal of Nursing Education*.

Dr. Caputi is the editor of the *Innovation Column* in the National League for Nursing's journal *Nursing Education Perspectives*, is a Certified Nurse Educator, was inducted as a fellow into the NLN's Academy of Nursing Education, and has served on the NLN's Board of Governors as well as numerous task forces and committees for the NLN. She is currently a site visitor for the NLN's Commission for Nursing Education Accreditation (CNEA).

For more information, current news, and teaching tools,
please visit Dr. Caputi's website at:
www.LindaCaputi.com

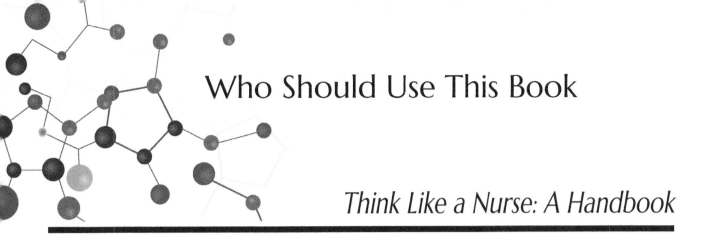

Who Should Use This Book

Think Like a Nurse: A Handbook

This book is written as a textbook for use in all levels of pre-licensed nursing education: LPN/LVN, Associate Degree, Baccalaureate Degree, and entry-level Master's Degree students. It can also be used in all RN to BSN programs as students revisit the process of **developing** clinical judgment then **applying** it to community health settings and management in the healthcare setting. RN to BSN students can also use this information as they are working with nursing students or orienting new staff in the practice setting. This book is also an excellent resource for nursing professional development practitioners and nurse preceptors as they work with new graduates and new nurse hires to expand their application of thinking as a staff nurse.

Finally, this book is a critical element for all students enrolled in Master's in Nursing Education programs. Those being educated as faculty in nursing programs and as nursing professional development practitioners must focus on teaching thinking if we all are to meet the ultimate goal of improved patient outcomes through excellent nursing care.

Please Note:
The tools and activities in this book are for individual use by the person purchasing the book.
Any further use, reproduction, or distribution for use by others is prohibited.

For students to use these tools and activities each student must have their own copy of the book.

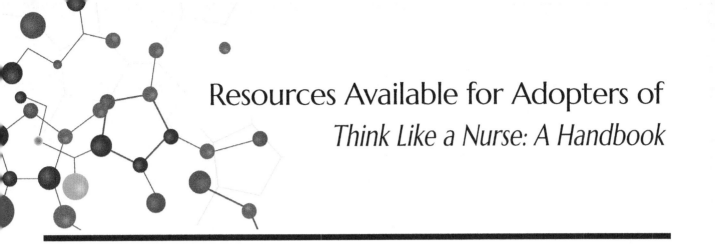

Resources Available for Adopters of
Think Like a Nurse: A Handbook

Teaching Resources for Nursing School/Program Faculty

Upon adopting *Think Like a Nurse: A Handbook* as a required student textbook, with the first order placed through the publisher, please contact Dr. Linda Caputi at LindaJCaputi@gmail.com. At that time Dr. Caputi will provide the faculty resources that accompany the book. These include:

- An overall general plan for integrating *Think Like a Nurse: A Handbook* into a nursing curriculum.

- Six steps for teaching each thinking skill.

- A topical weekly outline for integrating *Think Like a Nurse: A Handbook* into a course.

- Weekly lesson plans for a full semester course that include lesson objectives, teaching strategies/learning activities, homework assignments, in-class activities, and ideas and directions for using case studies to apply the thinking skills learned.

- One-hour free phone consultation with Dr. Caputi to discuss how you can use *Think Like a Nurse: A Handbook* in your nursing program.

Nursing Professional Development Practitioners

Nursing Professional Development Practitioners can use *Think Like a Nurse: A Handbook* in their onboarding/nurse orientation/residency programs. Ensuring new nursing hires can engage in clinical judgment to ensure safe patient care and improve patient outcomes is an overall goal of all healthcare environments. The above resources available for nursing schools are also available to Nursing Professional Development Practitioners. However, there are additional resources in the form of online modules available for purchase that can be incorporated into your orientation/residency programs for both Preceptors and New Hires. Please contact Dr. Caputi at LindaJCaputi@gmail.com for more information.

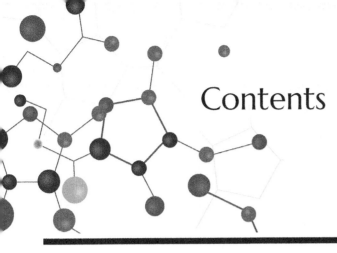

Contents

Think Like a Nurse: A Handbook

CHAPTER 1

Why this Book and Why Do Nurses Need to Learn about Critical Thinking?

You may be asking: Why this book? Don't I already know how to critically think?

Yes, you likely do know how to use critical thinking. However, adults typically do not think about their thinking and specifically explain to themselves the steps they are taking to solve a problem. Your thinking has become automatic.

The purpose of this book is to bring to your awareness the steps you take when solving problems in your everyday life. Once that is reviewed and you become consciously aware of the processes you use to make decisions, those thinking skills are then applied to nursing. The overall purpose of this book is to teach you how to use thinking in nursing for the purpose of providing safe, quality patient care; improving patient outcomes; and improving the healthcare environment in which you work. The *Future of Nursing* (IOM, 2011) report reminded us that nurses not only do nursing, but they also improve nursing. Engaging in nursing practice and improving nursing both require critical thinking.

Critical thinking applied to nursing is termed clinical judgment or clinical reasoning. There are other terms sometimes used, but these two terms are commonly used. Before nurses can apply clinical judgment/clinical reasoning to patient care and healthcare situations they **must first develop clinical judgment/clinical reasoning**. This book does just that—helps you **develop** clinical judgment/clinical reasoning then provides practice **applying** clinical judgment/clinical reasoning to nursing. The first step of **developing** clinical judgment/clinical reasoning is often missing in nursing education. This book was written to fill that critical need.

Why Learning to Think is a Critical Piece of your Nursing Education

Healthcare settings are very dynamic environments; circumstances can change often and very quickly. These settings are often unpredictable. The unexpected can happen without much warning (Levett-Jones, 2010). The nurse must be ready to respond by immediately using clinical judgment/clinical reasoning that is required to deal with the situation.

Patients often display manifestations that indicate their condition is worsening. The alert and thinking nurse recognizes these manifestations and intervenes immediately. Unfortunately, this is not always the case and the warning signs of impending deterioration are not recognized and treated (Purling & King, 2012). Patients can experience acute deterioration in their condition leading to longer hospital stays, unnecessary suffering, and even death.

Fortunately, most patients for whom you will care follow a typical path to recovery. The care they require is predictable and manageable by the well-informed nurse. However, you may care for patients who experience an unexpected occurrence, complications, or pre-existing conditions that complicate their recovery. Even the patient who appears to be recovering well can experience a sudden change in condition. The nurse must be prepared to recognize early, and often subtle, signs of an unexpected change in the patient's condition so interventions can be implemented. If interventions are not implemented, the patient may continue to deteriorate. If the patient dies, this is known as "failure to rescue."

An additional issue that contributes to poor patient outcomes is the unfortunate reality of errors. Many patients become very ill and even die because of errors made by medical personnel (Makary & Daniel, 2016). These errors are often the result of poor thinking processes.

Noting this reality in health care so early in this book is not to frighten you, but rather to impress upon you why learning how to think is equally important as learning nursing knowledge/content and psychomotor skills. Learning to think like a nurse with lots of practice activities to guide your thinking helps you gain the skills and confidence to identify patients in need of help and to improve patient outcomes. Preparation for this aspect of nursing practice provides what you need to care for patients and ensure their safety. It helps to make you practice ready.

Critical Thinking

An initial question to consider is: "What is critical thinking?" There are many terms used in nursing to represent thinking including critical thinking, clinical reasoning, clinical judgment, clinical decision making, and others. This book uses the term critical thinking to refer to general thinking and problem solving used in everyday life. The terms clinical reasoning or clinical judgment are used when applying critical thinking to nursing practice. These terms are used interchangeably in this book. The nursing program in which you are enrolled or from which you graduated may have used other terms related to thinking. Whatever term a nursing program uses, it is important the term is defined, and the teaching of thinking is taught in a systematic, organized manner across the curriculum.

> **Critical thinking:** logical and realistic thoughtful judgments that are directed toward clarifying what is true and what is false (Ennis, 1987, in Cannon & Boswell, 2016, p. 18).

> **Clinical judgment/clinical reasoning:** the thinking nurses use to make judgments about a patient situation. It is a logical process of collecting cues, processing information, understanding the problem or situation, then planning and implementing interventions. The final

steps in clinical judgment include evaluating the outcomes of the thinking and reflecting on the thinking process itself. The purpose of reflection is to learn from the situation to grow in the ability to use clinical reasoning (Levett-Jones, 2010).

Everyday Thinking Versus Thinking in Nursing

In everyday life, the thinking used is what is known as simplistic or ordinary thinking. This type of thinking includes guessing, assuming, or just believing something without examining supportive evidence or analyzing data to determine a course of action. This type of thinking may be all that is needed in many everyday interactions (Erickson & Lanning, 2014). However, when dealing with patients and events in the healthcare environment, simplistic thinking isn't a safe or acceptable form of thinking.

The type of critical thinking used by the nurse is **deliberate, skillful, responsible, and thoughtful**. Nurses use a deliberate process for engaging in critical thinking in their professional roles. However, it is important to note at this time that if you were to ask nurses about the deliberate process behind their thinking, it is likely most nurses will not be able to explain their step-by-step thinking that led them to a conclusion. This is because most nurses in practice are at the expert level of functioning. Experts use intuitive thinking and no longer delineate or recall each step of their thinking process. Their thinking becomes automatic.

Nurses base their thinking on criteria that are relevant to the situation, evidence, and standards that support the thinking process. The purpose of this book is to teach you how to learn about and use this type of thinking. The book provides a framework and a language for you to use to communicate your thinking to others.

A basic assumption of this book is that critical thinking can be taught. Most nursing students know how to engage in critical thinking. The issue is they may not realize the type of thinking they are using to solve everyday problems is actually critical thinking. This book presents examples of thinking from everyday life to provide evidence of thinking the student is currently using. It then teaches students how to apply that type of thinking to nursing situations, both with patients and to handle problems in the healthcare

> The type of critical thinking used by the nurse is deliberate, skillful, responsible, and thoughtful.

environment. This approach connects your old way of thinking to a new application of that thinking to demonstrate that thinking in nursing uses the same thinking skills and strategies you may already possess, but they are used within a nursing context.

This book can help you learn to think like a nurse and move you through the stages of thinking on your path to higher level thinking. The book provides many examples and activities for you to apply your thinking to nursing. Nursing and healthcare are very complex worlds; a step-by-step method for learning to think like a nurse will help you navigate through this complexity to make decisions that support safe, quality care and improve patient outcomes.

Characteristics or Factors that Affect Critical Thinking

At this point it may be helpful to list some characteristics or factors that affect critical thinking.

1. Nursing students and nurses think the way they were taught to think.

2. Before students can be asked to "use critical thinking" they must first learn what critical thinking is and learn how critical thinking is applied in nursing.

3. Reflection on decisions made is important to improve thinking. People do not learn by experience alone, but by reflecting on and thinking about their experiences (Cannon & Boswell, 2016).

4. Good clinical judgment requires the nurse to look at the situation within the total patient picture rather than as an isolated issue.

5. Sound clinical judgment requires knowledge of the patient and the patient's situation which is also known as contextual thinking—applying thinking to the specific patient or health-care situation.

6. The clinical decisions that are made are dependent on the healthcare setting in which they occur (Cappelletti, Engel, & Prentice, 2014).

7. Clinical judgments are more influenced by the ability of the nurse to think about a situation than by the objective information related to the situation. That is, the nurse must be able to determine what information is meaningful and how to use that information to make a decision (Tanner, 2006).

8. Educational strategies that teach critical thinking and engage students in using critical thinking are necessary requirements to learning to think like a nurse.

9. Effective clinical decision making is necessary for positive patient outcomes (Cappelletti, Engel, & Prentice, 2014).

10. Nurses use self-guided thinking when making decisions.

Self-Guided Thinking

Self-guided thinkers are independent thinkers who are able to explain their thinking, determine what thinking needs to be employed in a particular situation, then apply their thinking to arrive at a sound decision. A major goal of this book is to help you become a self-guided thinker. This book provides what you need to "internalize" a thinking process, but you will need to put forth the effort and motivation to learn and use the process taught. Basically, learning requires time and effort (Nilson, 2013).

This book provides lots of practice activities. It is important that you use these activities, gather information, engage in thinking, review your work, present your work to your teacher/preceptor, and request feedback. This feedback is also known as debriefing. Debriefing is a critical conversation between you and your teacher/preceptor which provides a critique about your thinking. This debriefing feedback reinforces your correct thinking and clarifies any misconceptions you may have. Debriefing is critical to your learning. These practice activities are mandatory to developing thinking skills. It is important to realize that just reading this book, even if you read it over and over, does not mean you know how to think. You must actually engage in the thinking activities to:

1. Learn what you still need to learn about thinking even if you believe you understand when reading the book. Compare learning to think to learning a nursing psychomotor skill such as hanging an intravenous bag of fluids. You can read about that skill over and over, but you do not know if you can actually perform that skill if you never hang an IV bag of fluids. Additionally, the more IV bags you hang, the more skillful you become. This same explanation applies to learning thinking skills. If you don't complete the activities in this book that guide your thinking you will not know if you can actually engage in the thinking required of a nurse.

2. Solidify the process into your long term memory. The more you engage in thinking the better thinker you will become.

Nilson (2013) conducted a literature search about the benefits of self-guided thinking (also known as self-regulated learning) and found this type of learning with deliberate practice enhances:

1. Student performance/achievement

2. The amount and depth of student thinking

3. Students' conscious focus on their learning

4. The development of reflective and responsible professionalism

These findings are exactly what is needed in nursing education. Many students, and even graduates in their first nursing position, are not aware of the thinking processes they use. Being a self-guided thinker means you are consciously aware of your thinking. Your thinking is a planned process not a "hit or miss" process. Critical thinking is not magical or mysterious, although when talking with an expert it may appear to be. On many occasions when I hear an expert speak, I wonder how that person was able to use the knowledge of the field and arrive at such as conclusion. I am truly impressed. I often think that person must possess some superhuman power. However, the reality is that person was able to engage in thinking at a very high level to arrive at that conclusion. That high level thinking was achieved by first learning how to think and practice thinking on many occasions and in a variety of contexts. In other words, **deliberate practice with contextual thinking**.

Deliberate Practice

Deliberate practice is the beginning point to achieving expert performance (Nilson, 2013). The path to expert thinking requires many instances of deliberate practice, breaking down all the elements of thinking that must be used to reach a sound decision. As you engage in deliberate practice you will constantly reflect on the thinking you used, identify what went right, identify any errors, correct the errors, then use what you learned for the next deliberate practice session. The activities in this book provide a means for the deliberate practice you need to unpack thinking, learn all the thinking processes, use them, then reflect on your thinking to learn from any mistakes.

Self-guided thinkers engage in self-assessment. Self-assessment is critical for growth and maturation as a thinker. This requires learners to be responsible for learning how to think and to grow as a thinker. This is known as having an "internal locus of control". The location of the control for learning lies within the learner. The teacher/preceptor are important sources of feedback, but the learner must be internally motivated to learn.

Your teacher or preceptor is part of this process. They can help you reflect on your thinking to identify and correct your errors in thinking and provide guidance. This reflection is a critical part of the process. We learn by experience, not necessarily because of the experience, but by reflecting on the experience. This approach works for new learners as well as experienced nurses.

> With deliberate practice, you will demonstrate connections among many pieces of information and discover solutions to problems by applying critical thinking abilities to nursing.

Deliberate practice is not easy work. Deliberate practice is hard work that requires repetition, over and over. This is mentally demanding and can be emotionally draining, but it is necessary. The reward of better patient outcomes is worth the effort. Again, compare learning to think to learning a psychomotor skill. Repeated practice is required to perfect the skill. When caring for patients, students request to perform as many psychomotor skills as possible because they realize the more times they perform a skill the better they will become at performing that skill. This truth also applies to learning to be a good thinker. You must have time to describe your thinking, practice thinking, and demonstrate thinking before being assessed on how well you've learned thinking. With deliberate practice, you will demonstrate connections among many pieces of information and discover solutions to problems by applying critical thinking abilities to nursing. You will do this all within a specific patient context explaining how your decision may change depending on the patient. Critical thinking and clinical reasoning are important to transform the nursing information you are learning to useable knowledge, **not just learning information but using information for the best possible decision**. Deliberate practice provides opportunities to become an excellent thinker in nursing.

There is a major difference between learning and perfecting a psychomotor skill and learning and perfecting thinking skills. A psychomotor skill is one discrete task. Learning thinking is much more complex with many variables and factors that may not be obvious to the nurse. However, learning to think like a nurse is possible and should start on the first day of your first nursing course.

Contextual Thinking

A major component of critical thinking in any situation is to always consider the context in which the situation is occurring. This is called **contextual thinking**. You will learn many normal values, guidelines, and general information about nursing practice and patient care. But just as you consider the context when making a decision in your everyday life, you will consider the context in which the nursing situation occurs. Let's look at an example from everyday life. Teens typically have a curfew by which time they need to be home. A curfew time for a teen may be 11 PM on Friday and Saturday evenings. On a particular Saturday evening, the teen does not arrive home until 1 AM. Her parents greet her at the door, say good-night, and retire to bed as does the teen. There are no problems or issues with the 1 AM time. Looking at the situation by simply applying the rule, one would likely conclude the parents must not have been aware of the time. But they were. The difference is that on this evening there was a special dance at the school that did not end until 12:30 AM. Therefore, the rule was changed for this evening. In this context the teen returned home on time. Not knowing the context of this situation, it might appear the parents did not act responsibility; however, considering the context the parent's behavior is acceptable.

This is a very simple example but demonstrates the importance of context. This is an important consideration when making decisions in nursing practice and is an overall guideline nurses use in all decision making—**consider the context**.

> The overall purpose of
> this book is to teach you
> how to use thinking in nursing
> for the purpose of providing
> safe, quality patient care;
> improving patient outcomes;
> and improving the healthcare
> environment in which
> you work.

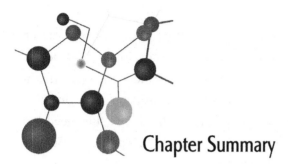

Chapter Summary

In summary, the purpose of this book is to offer an evidence-based approach to teaching clinical reasoning in nursing because educational strategies influence what a nurse brings to the situation. It is difficult, if not impossible, for the student nurse to make sound clinical decisions if learning to think like a nurse was not part of the planned nursing curriculum.

CHAPTER 2

The Caputi Model for Teaching Thinking in Nursing

Students want to be nurses. They see what nurses do and hear what nurses say about medical diagnoses and how to care for patients from the medical model perspective. They want to perform as many psycho-motor skills as possible. Students cannot see nurses think so may be unaware of the complex thinking that underlies what they see nurses do. They do not hear, nor do they see, how nurses engage in thinking. Nurses think through and solve dozens of problems every day. Many of the problems solved relate to patient care. However, many other problems nurses solve relate to the healthcare environment, interactions with other healthcare providers, constant interruptions, and a host of other issues. Because students cannot see the mental processes in which nurses constantly engage throughout the day, they may not understand the importance of how complicated these thinking processes can be.

This book and the Caputi Model help you to uncover and unpack the thinking processes nurses use. The book presents a systematic, formalized approach to learn thinking across the curriculum. Critical thinking must be unpacked and made clear through specific language that is deliberately taught and used if it is to be valued (Rubenfeld & Scheffer, 2015). You may be asked by your teacher to use critical thinking or to explain your thinking. Without formal education in using thinking, students often attempt to address the teacher's request without actually knowing how to think, or how to explain their thinking, mainly because they have not learned how to think in nursing situations. You must learn specific thinking processes to enable you to articulate your thinking.

> Nurses think through and solve dozens of problems every day. Many of the problems solved relate to patient care.

Three Components of Learning Clinical Judgment/Clinical Reasoning

Unpacking clinical reasoning begins with identifying its components. The Caputi Model for Teaching Thinking in Nursing (Caputi, 2016) was developed in 2011 after years of studying the literature on thinking in nursing and applying that research to teach students to think like a nurse. This model presents an approach for learning clinical judgment/clinical reasoning using specific language that unpacks thinking.

Students learn to use this language as they approach problem solving in all learning environments. The three components of the Caputi Model for Teaching Thinking in Nursing are:

- Dr. Benner's Novice to Expert Theory (Benner, 2001)

- Dr. Tanner's Clinical Judgment Model (Tanner, 2006)

- Specific critical thinking skills and strategies

These three components overlap to provide a structure for learning clinical judgment/clinical reasoning in nursing:

Component 1
Dr. Benner's Novice to Expert Theory

Dr. Benner's model describes the stages of developing nurses as they become experts in their practice. This model covers 5 stages. The nursing student should accomplish the first two stages while enrolled in a nursing program.

When you enter a nursing program as a student you are considered in the Novice Stage. You arrive with no experience of nursing situations within the scope of practice you are studying. Teachers deconstruct all the nursing content by putting it into simpler, out of context terms so you can understand what is being taught. As a novice, you learn specific rules to follow and apply those rules to all situations, regardless of context. Your practice is rule-based. An example of a rule is, "The normal blood pressure is 120/80."

Your teacher may share with you at this beginning level that nursing is not black or white, but grey. We, as teachers, must explain what is meant by grey. Grey really means, "It depends." The "it depends" answer requires situational (contextual) thinking, not rule-based thinking. That is, you must consider how you will use the rule you learned within the context of the specific patient situation. For example, you compare the patient's blood pressure to the rule of 120/80. However, a much higher or lower blood pressure may be acceptable depending on the situation. This is the "it depends" part. The "it depends" requires consideration of the patient's situation, or the context. Providing deliberate practice using a rule in a contextual manner is one of the major purposes of this book.

During the first semester of nursing courses, teachers demonstrate to students how the rules they are learning are applied to a patient considering all aspects of the patient situation. Then the nurse makes a decision. Students learn that simply applying a rule to all situations without considering the context of the patient leads to faulty thinking and poor decisions. Although novices are able to readily identify patient data, they are unable to identify important cues, especially as the complexity of a situation increases. The novice applies the rule regardless of the situation in large part due to an inability to differentiate what is important from what is not important (Koharchik, Caputi, Robb, & Culleiton, 2015).

> The 5 Stages of
> Dr. Benner's
> Novice to Expert Theory
>
> *Novice Stage*
> *Advanced Beginner Stage*
> *Competent Stage*
> *Proficient Stage*
> *Expert Stage*

Once you learn the "grey" lesson by applying rules within a variety of patient contexts and in a variety of healthcare environments, you are ready to be guided into the Advanced Beginner Stage of Benner's skill acquisition model. In this stage you encounter additional experiences using rules in real and/or simulated situations to move from simple rules to guide your behavior to applying principles to guide your actions. You practice applying rules and learning about aspects of a situation that are relevant and aspects of a situation that are not relevant based on the specific patient situation. As you work through these types of experiences, you begin to use clinical reasoning based on the specifics of a situation; that is, decisions made and actions taken become situation driven rather than rule driven.

At this point it is helpful to use learning activities that provide opportunities to apply rules to individual patient situations. This book provides those learning activities. You will compare and contrast patients with similar conditions to discover individual patient nuances (patient specific differences) that contribute to situational thinking rather than rule based thinking. In so doing, you begin to learn differences among patients who appear similar, but are quite different based on the specifics of the patient context.

The last three stages of Dr. Benner's Novice to Expert Theory are completed after graduating from nursing school and entering the nursing profession. These stages are competent, proficient, and expert. It takes approximately five years working in a profession to achieve the expert level.

Component 2
Dr. Tanner's Clinical Judgment Model

The second component of the Caputi Model for Teaching Thinking in Nursing is Dr. Tanner's Clinical Judgment Model (Tanner, 2006). The Clinical Judgment Model breaks down thinking into four steps:

- Noticing
- Interpreting
- Responding
- Reflecting

These four steps represent the thinking process used by nurses. Although the steps are described as separate, distinct steps, these steps do not always flow in a linear fashion. That is, the nurse may notice something about a patient situation that represents a real or potential problem then interpret that situation as an issue. However, during the interpreting stage, the nurse may return to the noticing step to collect additional information to more clearly understand and define the problem.

Another way to interpret these steps is to put them in the form of questions such as:

- What did I notice?
- What does it mean?
- What will I do?
- What was the effect of what I did and of my thinking?

This book uses these steps to organize the thinking skills nurses use. However, keep in mind that many of the thinking skills may be used in steps other than the ones under which they are listed in this book. This book lists the thinking skills and strategies under the step where the skill is most likely used, keeping in mind the skill may be used in other steps as well. This provides a structured approach for "unpacking" clinical reasoning in nursing for learning purposes.

*~Following is a brief explanation of each of the
four steps of the Tanner Clinical Judgment Model~*

NOTICING

The Noticing Step involves collecting data about the patient or a healthcare situation. The nurse uses assessment techniques such as observation and auscultation to collect data. Additionally, an important skill to use during noticing is thoughtful questioning used to explore all aspects of the situation. During the Noticing Step the nurse notices that something is different than what was expected. Something doesn't seem right. For example, the nurse assesses the patient and collects new information that was not included in the report received from the nurse on the previous shift. Or, perhaps the nurse has learned the typical presentation of a patient with a particular medical diagnosis, but the current patient demonstrates a variation from what was expected.

Because nurses also face issues and problems in the healthcare environment, this is also an aspect of nursing that sometimes requires attention. Consider the following scenario. There are several occurrences throughout the nurse's shift when the medications delivered from the pharmacy are not the ones that were ordered for the patient. This is a problem that needs to be addressed so a wrong medication is not administered to the patient. This is a problem with the environment in which the nurse works. The nurse must bring attention to the problem and work to correct it. Nurses not only engage in nursing, but they also work to improve nursing. The safety of the healthcare environment is basic to safe patient care.

There are some factors that affect what the nurse notices. The level of the nurse's knowledge is important. In your the first nursing course you may not notice patient or healthcare environmental issues because of your unfamiliarity with nursing. With each passing week you learn more, and you become more prepared to notice issues that must be addressed.

Personal characteristics of the nurse also influence what is noticed (Nielsen & Lasater, 2017). You may enter nursing with many preconceived ideas and attitudes about a number of issues that can affect patient care. These preconceived ideas and attitudes greatly influence your ability to notice. For example, if the student believes that all elderly people are confused, then a patient's confusion may go unnoticed.

The nurse must have the self-confidence to be comfortable asking for help. Not noticing a problem or issue because the nurse may need help with the situation is an unacceptable behavior. Often times something just doesn't seem right but the nurse may be unable to identify or define the nature of the problem. The nurse must be comfortable asking for help and never leave a potential problem unnoticed; that is, unidentified.

The more experiences you have with a specific patient, the more keen your noticing ability becomes. That is, what may **not** be typical for patients in a particular situation, may be typical for a patient based on that individual patient situation. The greater the familiarity with a patient, the more enabled you are to know what is normal and what is not normal for the patient.

> The nurse must have the self-confidence to be comfortable asking for help. Not noticing a problem or issue because the nurse may need help with the situation is an unacceptable behavior.

Another factor that influences noticing is the context or environment of care (Nielsen & Lasater, 2017). For example, a laboratory value may be acceptable for a patient with a chronic illness in a long-term care environment, but the same laboratory value may not be acceptable for an acutely ill patient with no pre-existing illnesses admitted to the acute care hospital.

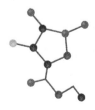

As would be expected, the more you learn about nursing and the more experiences you have providing nursing care, the more astute your *noticing* will become.

INTERPRETING

Once you notice there is a problem and collect data, you must make sense of that information. You interpret what the data mean. An overall term for all the thinking skills in this step is **data analysis**. Nurses analyze the data using a variety of thinking skills and strategies to make sense of the data to determine issues, problems, or concerns.

This is a unique step in the process; that is, your interpretation is dependent on a variety of factors that influenced what you noticed. The thoughtful questioning you used during the Noticing Step is helpful at this point because you now use that information to explore possibilities and alternatives for care, or solutions to a problem based on the individual patient context.

The way the information is interpreted can differ depending on the individual nurse's background, the healthcare environment, and the specifics about the patient. Because of these variables, how the information is interpreted varies among nurses. It is most important that you interpret information correctly so the actions you plan will be what is needed in the specific situation (Nielsen & Lasater, 2017).

This is a very important step because the conclusions at which you arrive based on the data you collect, determine actions you will or will not take for the patient or to solve a healthcare environment problem. It is important to identify the salient (important) factors that define the problem. At this point you recall the rules, or general guidelines, you learned in your nursing courses, then apply them within the context of the problem identified. The rules or guidelines will not be strictly or absolutely applied; rather, the salient aspects specific to the situation determine how that rule or guideline will be applied.

Again, the more practice you have applying these rules and guidelines, the better you will become in knowing how much ambiguity (wiggle room) you have with the rule/guideline.

RESPONDING

The conclusions you made based on interpretation of the data determine how you will respond to the situation. In other words, the determinations made in the Interpreting Step are important for deciding how and to what degree you will respond. For example, based on your thinking in the first two steps, you may determine a possible problem can be addressed by ambulating the patient. However, how far and for how long you will ambulate the patient is affected by the factors related to the patient situation as identified in the interpreting stage. That is, you may decide to impose limitations related to the ambulation activity based on the specific patient's condition. You may determine that one patient may only be able to ambulate a few feet, while another patient can ambulate much further. Making this determination is critical for safe care.

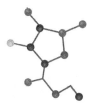

The determinations made in the Interpreting Step are important for deciding how and to what degree you will *respond*, which is critical for safe care.

REFLECTING

Reflecting on your thinking occurs in this step. As mentioned previously, reflective thinking is tantamount to learning and growing as a nurse. Reviewing your thinking and its effectiveness encourages deeper understanding of your ability to think, supports self-evaluation, and, with honest reflection, fosters growth in your ability to use critical thinking and clinical judgment. There are two types of reflection that occur in this step.

Reflection-IN-Action

Reflection-in-action occurs while you are providing care for the patient or addressing the healthcare environment issue. In the case of patient care, as you are performing a nursing intervention you continue to collect cues from the patient that tell you what you are doing is or isn't working; or, what you are doing needs to be modified for this particular patient. Reflection-in-action is happening in real time, as you are providing care. Because of the ambiguous and sometimes quickly changing patient condition or unexpected happening, the nurse must always consider how the patient is responding to the planned intervention while carrying out that intervention. For example, you plan to ambulate the patient to the nurse's station and back. However, halfway to that goal, the patient becomes dizzy. You will immediately revise your plan.

Reflection-ON-Action

As the name implies, reflection-on-action occurs upon completion of the action. This step is critical to improving thinking. During this step you mentally review what just happened to determine what went right and what went wrong. What you learn from the experience is used to improve your thinking abilities and your nursing knowledge base. This is the actual learning from experience step. Without this reflection it is difficult to learn from your experiences. As you engage in reflective practice throughout your nursing program and throughout your nursing career, you will continue on your path toward the Expert Stage of Dr. Benner's Novice to Expert Theory.

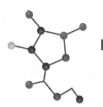

Reflective thinking is tantamount to learning and growing as a nurse.

Activity

Consider the Clinical Judgment Model. This type of thinking is not exclusive to nursing. You have worked through these same steps in your everyday life to solve problems. You probably have made judgments such as:

- Judgments in the workplace

- Judgments about parenting

- Judgments about fashion

- Judgments about yard work

- Judgments about life style choices: exercising, type of diet, smoking, drinking alcohol, etc.

Here is an example of using this decision making model in everyday life.

BRIEF EXPLANATION OF PROBLEM:
A friend stops by and is very upset. She is crying because she needs a dress for an unexpected occasion, but can't afford to buy one.

STEP IN THE MODEL	EXPLANATION OF THIS STEP IN SOLVING THE PROBLEM
Noticing: *Gather data*	What you know about this person: She works hard; saves money; helps her family as much as she can.
Interpreting: *Make sense of the information*	You know this person and how she may react because of past experiences, so you use this information as you plan your response. You decide to buy the dress for her and let her decide how she will pay you back.
Responding: *Take action*	You carry out the planned actions → individualized for this friend based on what you know of the situation and know of her. You lend her the money for the dress.
Reflecting: *Evaluate and learn from the experience*	Reflection in action—you changed your approach slightly based on her response during your conversation and offered her an additional month to pay back the loan.
	Reflection on action—You review in your mind how the exchange occurred and determine it went well. However, you know that in the future you may need other alternatives for repayment of the loan.

The next table presents a similar situation but is somewhat different. That is, the context is a little different.

BRIEF EXPLANATION OF PROBLEM:

A friend stops by and is very upset. She also needs a dress for an unexpected occasion, but can't afford to buy one. She knows you are very supportive of your friends and asks if you can lend her the money.

STEP IN THE MODEL	EXPLANATION OF THIS STEP IN SOLVING THE PROBLEM
Noticing: *Gather data*	What you know about this person: She spends money every day and doesn't save. She is known to borrow from others and often times does not repay them or only repays them if the lender makes frequent requests.
Interpreting: *Make sense of the information*	This friend has a recurring problem that is self-imposed so providing money each time she asks is not a good solution. Teaching the friend how to help herself would be more helpful.
Responding: *Take action*	Explain to the friend that you are unable to lend her money at this time. Offer to teach her about how to budget her money so she can be prepared for unexpected occasions.
Reflecting: *Evaluate and learn from the experience*	Although the friend is upset that you won't lend her money, she has a recurring problem that is self-imposed so providing money each time is not a good solution. Teaching the friend how to help herself would be more helpful. She did not accept the offer to help her budget her money, but at this time you believe this was still the best option for this friend. Your friend decides to wear a dress she had previously purchased but had never worn, eliminating the need to buy a new one.

In the table below provide an example how you have used these steps to solve a problem in your life. This does not have to be a big problem, but can be one of the many situations you face and must resolve on a daily basis. Think through your experience and determine which actions align with each of the steps in the model.

BRIEF EXPLANATION OF PROBLEM:	
STEP IN THE MODEL	EXPLANATION OF THIS STEP IN SOLVING THE PROBLEM
Noticing: *Gather data*	
Interpreting: *Make sense of the information*	
Responding: *Take action*	
Reflecting: *Evaluate and learn from the experience*	

Developing this ability to reflect and use the results of your reflective thinking to improve your thinking continues throughout your nursing career. Because the healthcare environment is ever changing and patients are different in so many ways, your learning to think never ceases. Therefore, you must develop this process and become a reflective practitioner. Remember, do not just reflect on negative results. Nurses often focus on negative outcomes and work to determine how to improve (Nielsen & Lasater, 2017). That is a critical piece of reflection. However, so is reflection on your positive results. It is important to contemplate how what you did worked well in the situation and how it might be used or perhaps revised based on the context of future patients.

Component 3
Critical Thinking Skills and Strategies

The third component of the Caputi Model for Teaching Thinking in Nursing is a listing of specific critical thinking skills and strategies. Breaking down critical thinking into its parts means teaching students **specific** critical thinking skills and strategies. Learning these thinking skills and strategies and applying them to nursing is fundamental. Unfortunately, this is often the missing piece for many nursing programs (Caputi, 2010a; Caputi, 2010b). These skills and strategies provide the verbiage you need to track your thinking then explain your thinking. You may have discovered the answer to a question using critical thinking, but you cannot articulate how you arrived at the answer because you have not specifically learned the thinking skills and strategies you used to address the question. This is because you do not have the knowledge base related to thinking skills that is needed to answer the question and explain your thinking. This book provides that information as well as practice using those thinking skills and strategies.

Without a knowledge base about thinking, you are not able to apply metacognition, which is what your teacher/preceptor is asking you to do with many different questions, such as, "Why will you implement that nursing action?" or "Why was that procedure ordered?". Metacognition refers to your ability to think about your thinking. Metacognition refers to your ability to understand your thinking, control your thinking processes, and explain your thinking.

There are many critical thinking skills and strategies nurses use. It is critical you learn these thinking skills so you are able to explain your thinking and apply metacognition, thinking about your thinking. This critical piece is often missing in teaching students to think like a nurse. This book provides specific guidance applying thinking skills in clinical situations. In the nursing education literature there are many critical thinking skills identified (Caputi, 2010a; Caputi, 2010b; Lasater, 2011; Paul & Elder, 2014). The following chapters in this book present these thinking skills and strategies and provide activities you can use to apply them to nursing.

You must not only learn what these are but must actually use them in clinical situations. Through this process you learn what is meant by "nursing is not black or white, but grey".

Putting the Three Components Together

None of the individual components alone can result in learning how to think like a nurse. They all work together to build thinking across time. You will use the four steps of Tanner's Clinical Judgment Model to organize your thinking then use critical thinking skills when working through each step of the model.

As you become skilled using thinking skills by applying Tanner's Clinical Judgment Model, you will move through Benner's Novice Stage entering the Advanced Beginner Stage. The very deliberate practice assignments that require you to apply thinking to individual patient care and to deal with other nursing situations help you transition from Novice to Advanced Beginner. You move from rule-based thinking (Novice Stage) to situation-based thinking (Advanced Beginner Stage).

As a student you need an organized approach to learning when you enter a nursing program. Nursing is new and, perhaps, even foreign to you. Your program is likely designed to proceed from simple to complex, leveling content and nursing skills across the program. Initial learning is structured with simple relationships among concepts in theory and step-by-step guidelines for nursing skills. As you advance through the program, your performance of nursing skills and application of nursing knowledge become less rule-based and more situational. Your performance of nursing skills and application of theory should become less deliberate and more automatic.

This is the goal with teaching thinking. In the initial phases you learn the pieces of the three major components of the Caputi Model for Teaching Thinking in Nursing. As you apply your learning in clinical practice, thinking should become automatic rather than a deliberate step-by-step process. However, before automatic thinking is possible, you must learn and use the thinking skills and strategies.

Without learning the building blocks of thinking in nursing, you cannot think about your thinking but only hope your thinking is correct as you work to answer the "why" questions posed.

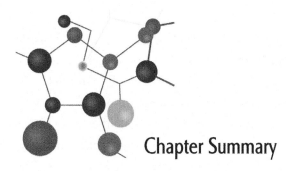

Chapter Summary

The Caputi Model for Teaching Thinking in Nursing is fairly simple. It is summarized as follows:

1. Learn individual critical thinking skills.

2. Engage in deliberate, focused practice applying each of the thinking skills in an actual clinical situation, a classroom clinical situation, or a simulation laboratory experience.

3. Demonstrate how what you are doing aligns with Tanner's evidence-based Clinical Judgment Model.

4. Demonstrate how you are progressing through the thinking of Benner's stages of Novice and Advanced Beginner.

5. Continue this process across the curriculum.

The end goal for implementing a deliberate approach to learning thinking is improved patient outcomes. As a new graduate applying for your first nursing position you must talk this talk. As you share in an interview all the psychomotor skills you performed while in the clinical setting throughout school, you should also share all the specific thinking skills you learned and how you applied them to identify potential complications, decrease the morbidity and mortality rate, decrease the failure to rescue rate, and improve patient outcomes. This is the ultimate goal of any nursing program.

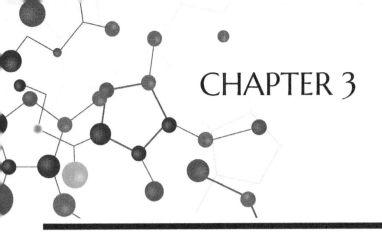

CHAPTER 3

Explanation of the
Following Chapters

This chapter explains the remaining chapters of the book.

CHAPTER 4

Chapter 4 teaches specific thinking skills and strategies of the Caputi Model for Teaching Thinking in Nursing. Each critical thinking skill is presented in the following format:

- The thinking skill is defined.
- An example of using that thinking skill in everyday life is presented.
- An explanation of how that thinking skill might be used in nursing is provided.

*The Tanner Clinical Judgment Model is used as an organizing structure
for application of the thinking skills.*

CHAPTER 5

Chapter 5 presents actual clinical activities. These are rather simple activities that provide step-by-step practice using each individual thinking skill in a nursing context. It is important to work through these activities in an actual clinical setting. **It is critical to note that nurses typically do not use one thinking skill at a time, but use many thinking skills to solve a problem.** However, applying these thinking skills one at a time allows careful study of the thinking process. That is, critical thinking is unpacked so you can learn how to think.

CHAPTER 6

Chapter 6 then provides more complex thinking activities. These more complex thinking activities require the use of a number of thinking skills applied to various patient situations.

CHAPTER 7

Chapter 7 expands the focus of the thinking activities to direct application to the healthcare setting and care in the community. These activities also require the use of a number of thinking skills applied to various healthcare settings.

Why These Activities?

Teachers continuously work to identify ways to teach nursing students how to think like a nurse. Most approaches require students to apply thinking to a variety of patient situations and problems in the health-care setting. The missing piece is teaching students the actual thinking process so they can **develop clinical judgment/clinical reasoning**. Many times students are asked to use thinking without learning about thinking in a simple, instructive manner. In other words, students must **develop** thinking skills before they can **use** thinking skills.

> Just learning the knowledge
> is never enough;
> knowing how to use
> that knowledge
> when needed in a
> specific situation
> is what nurses
> must be able to do.

So why the activities? Can't I just learn by reading the book? It is not enough to learn the knowledge presented in this book about thinking. Like all knowledge in nursing education, just knowing information does not always mean the nurse knows *how to use* the information when needed. Knowing how to use the information in an individual patient context is the basis for safe nursing care. Just learning the knowledge is never enough; knowing how to use that knowledge when needed in a specific situation is what nurses must be able to do. This is why practice with these thinking activities is so very much needed. This is the same as learning and perfecting psychomotor skills. You must practice, practice, practice! Applying thinking in a new discipline is not intuitive and automatic; it takes practice, practice, practice!

These practice thinking activities are critical to learning how to think. These activities can be viewed as scripts which are organized ways to approach a situation or a problem (Panadero, Alonso-Tapia, & Reche, 2013). This process is enhanced with well-designed, thoughtful questions and inquiries about thinking as you work through the activity (Lasater, 2011). Just as you learn a nursing psychomotor skill by reviewing the steps of the procedure and applying those steps during practice, learning how to think like a nurse is enhanced with a similar approach. However, that is not to say that you can memorize steps in thinking. What you are learning is an approach to thinking that can be applied to a variety of nursing situations. As the nurse, you must determine which thinking skills are needed to make decisions and solve patient problems. At first this process is very deliberate with careful thought throughout each step. However, the more practice you have with deliberate use of thinking skills, the more automatic your thinking in nursing becomes just as thinking in your everyday life is automatic. This is why practice using these thinking skills is so important. Just as with any skill, frequent deliberate practice leads to automatic, intuitive performance.

Consider driving a car. When you first learned to drive, you thought through each step, recalling and applying what you learned to the task of driving. The more you drove a motor vehicle, the more automatic your thinking became. You eventually developed the skill to the point where you drive your car intuitively without consciously thinking through each step. This same process applies to thinking in nursing.

A major strength of these activities is they all require you to not just work through the thinking but to reflect on that thinking. As mentioned earlier, learning from experience does not occur until you reflect on the experience. It is best to discuss reflection on your experience with your teacher/preceptor for maximum learning from these activities. Discussion (debriefing) with your teacher/preceptor about your work when completing these activities accelerates learning of clinical judgment/clinical reasoning (Hines & Wood, 2016). This guided, structured reflecting with subsequent debriefing with your teacher/preceptor may be the most important component when completing these activities leading to improved self-assessment and ability to think reflectively. The embedded cues and prompts enhance the learning process. The ultimate goal is you are able to apply this thinking process to new and different clinical situations as a self-guided thinker.

A Few Notes about the Activities

Prior to using these activities in the clinical setting, work with your teacher/preceptor to determine if there are any modifications he/she may want to make to the assignment.

In this book you are learning the **thinking processes** you will use when you apply nursing knowledge, perform psychomotor skills, and deal with situations related to the healthcare setting. As you work through these thinking activities in clinical situations, you are guided how to approach a specific situation, but you may need to locate additional information or may need assistance finding information to work through the activity. You may need to locate resources that provide the needed information about the situation at hand. Knowledge about sources of necessary information and how to access those sources is a critical piece of thinking in nursing.

Some of those sources include:

1. Your own previous learning

2. Your patient's medical record

3. Nursing textbooks

4. Online resources including reliable websites

5. Policy and procedure manuals

6. Published professional standards including your state nurse practice act providing information on scope of practice

7. Job descriptions

8. The nurse with whom you are working

9. Your teacher/preceptor

These are examples of sources of information. Other sources of information may be available depending on the situation. Access to scientific evidence (evidence-based nursing) from reliable sources is critical for making good decisions based on solid clinical judgment/clinical reasoning.

Suggestions to Strengthen Your Learning

As you work through the rest of this book, it is important to accept the basic educational fact that you are in charge of your learning. As a student you may often feel overwhelmed and struggle with how to learn. The following is a list of suggestions that are derived from current research about how people learn (Ambrose, et al, 2010; Brown, Roediger, & McDaniel, 2014). Please review these for they are important principles for learning that support use of these active learning activities as you learn to think like a nurse.

1. Learning is an inside job. As such, learning takes effort. You will soon come to realize that to learn something takes more than reading a book and listening to a teacher talk. Deep, durable learning—that is, learning that will serve you well in the future—takes active effort on your part.

2. Build on what you know; that is, link what you are learning to what you have already learned. Look for the commonalities and differences. Apply all you have learned to date to the situation at hand. Activities in this book will assist you with this task.

3. Building on what you know requires you to retrieve prior learning from your memory. Retrieving information from memory helps you know what you know and what you do not know; if you are having difficulty remembering something, you likely need to study that area a little more. Also, pulling information from your memory helps your brain strengthen your learning of that information which makes it easier for you to use that information in the future. For example, if you learned something in semester one but didn't use that information until semester four or until after you graduate, it will be difficult to recall that information. If, however, you are called upon to use that information in semesters two and three, recalling that same information in semester four or after you graduate will be much easier. This is critical for learning to think like a nurse.

4. To strengthen your thinking, you need time to think through and process your thinking. You then need time to reflect on your thinking to determine if your thinking was correct and to determine how you might improve your thinking. Give yourself time to engage in the thinking activities offered in this book.

5. Engaging in reflection also helps give meaning to new material by expressing it in your own words and connecting the new learning to what you already know. The more you can explain how your new learning connects to prior learning, the more connections you can make thus improving your grasp of new learning. These activities can help you make those connections.

6. The activities presented in the next chapters provide goal-directed practice; that is, the goal is to apply the components of the Caputi Model for Teaching Thinking in Nursing to learn to think like a nurse. Debriefing with your teacher/preceptor on your work is critical to enhance the quality of your learning.

7. These activities also provide opportunity for you to become a self-guided learner. Through these activities you can learn to monitor your own thinking and adjust your thinking as needed based on the patient situation or healthcare setting problem.

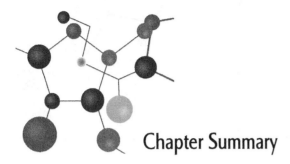

Chapter Summary

This chapter explained the purpose of the following chapters which contain the nuts and bolts of learning thinking.

Chapter 4 introduces and provides examples of the thinking skills and strategies taught in this book.

The remaining chapters provide activities for you to use to practice thinking in actual nursing situations. These activities are used starting in the first clinical nursing course then through all the remaining clinical courses to advance your level of thinking as a major component of practice readiness at the new graduate level.

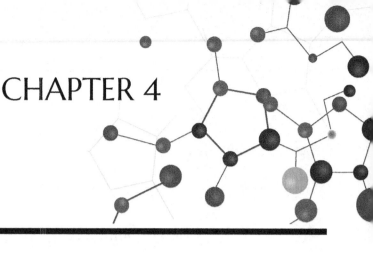

CHAPTER 4

Using Critical Thinking Skills and Strategies

This chapter presents thinking skills and strategies within the framework of the Tanner Clinical Judgment Model. All the thinking skills and strategies covered are listed under the four steps of the Tanner Clinical Judgment Model as described earlier in this book. It is important to understand that each of the thinking skills and strategies may be used in other steps than the one in which it is presented; however, for organizational and learning purposes the thinking skills and strategies that best align with a specific step are presented under that step.

The organization of content for each thinking skill and strategy presented in this chapter is as follows:

1. A definition of the thinking skill/strategy.

2. Example using that thinking skill/strategy in everyday life.

3. Example using that thinking skill/strategy in a nursing situation.

~Following is a list of thinking skills and strategies covered in this text~

Noticing

1. Identifying signs and symptoms

2. Assessing systematically and comprehensively

3. Gathering accurate information

4. Predicting potential complications

Interpreting

1. Clustering related information

2. Recognizing inconsistencies

3. Determining important information to collect

4. Distinguishing relevant from irrelevant information

5. Judging how much ambiguity is acceptable

6. Comparing and contrasting

7. Managing potential complications

8. Identifying assumptions

9. Setting priorities

10. Collaborating

Responding

1. Delegating

2. Communicating

3. Teaching others

Reflecting

1. Evaluating data

2. Evaluating and correcting thinking

Noticing Step

As discussed earlier, during the Noticing Step of clinical judgment, the nurse identifies areas of concern. However, what is noticed depends on:

1. The nurse's knowledge base

2. Personal characteristics of the nurse such as preconceived attitudes and self-confidence

3. Context: the individual patient situation or specific healthcare setting; that is, what is meaningful in one situation may not be meaningful in another

The nurse's knowledge base might include knowledge about diagnostic tests, the physiology of body systems, pathology of diseases, and concepts used in nursing practice. As you collect data during the Noticing Step of clinical judgment, think about and question your knowledge base.

*   What do you know?

*   What do you need to know? Are there holes in your knowledge base?

*   What information do you need to find out to address the problem?

*   What do you need to review in a reference book to determine the significance of the data you are collecting?

*   What sources of information will you use?

*   Are there any monitors or alarms in place that provide information about the patient's condition? Do you need to learn about this equipment?

Assessing your own knowledge base and identifying sources to augment that knowledge is an important activity prior to engaging in the thinking skills used to "notice."

Noticing, the first step of clinical judgment, forms the basis for the next steps of the thinking process. There are four thinking skills and strategies in the Noticing Step presented in this book:

1. Identifying signs and symptoms

2. Assessing systematically and comprehensively

3. Gathering complete and accurate data

4. Predicting potential complications

IDENTIFYING SIGNS AND SYMPTOMS

Definition

Signs and symptoms represent the objective and subjective data collected in a situation. In nursing, this thinking skill refers to an ability to identify aspects of a disease, side effects of a medication or other treatment/intervention, and a host of other factors that indicate the presence of an issue or problem for the patient. To identify signs and symptoms the nurse must have knowledge about all these factors as well as other information important to patient care such as safety, stress, and coping. Once signs and symptoms are identified they are compared to normal functioning and to the patient's previous assessment. This comparison helps the nurse make decisions about the information collected.

This thinking skill is constantly being used in the clinical setting. You will use this skill when performing your initial assessment of the patient, but also as you are working with the patient throughout the day to notice any early or subtle changes in the patient's condition. It is critical to use this skill for identifying changes in the patient's condition—no matter how subtle—because part of the nurse's responsibility is to notice changes that may indicate a worsening of the patient's condition and intervene before the situation becomes critical.

Before making decisions about information collected (Interpreting Step), the nurse must first know what to look for which is dependent on the three factors previously listed:

1. The nurse's knowledge base

2. Personal characteristics of the nurse such as preconceived attitudes and self-confidence

3. Context: the individual patient situation or the type of healthcare environment: acute care, long term care, clinic, medical office, etc.

Example Using "Identifying Signs and Symptoms" in Everyday Life

There are many times throughout the day when you collect signs and symptoms of a situation and compare that data to what you expect as the normal. For example:

> *One Friday evening you arrive home and find the following: kitchen is a mess with pizza boxes and remaining pizza on counter, soft drink cans in the sink, the television on, lights in every room on, and teen-age children in bed. Your normal expectations about the condition of the house are: kitchen clean, dishes from dinner put away, quiet house, teen-age children in bed, one light on in the living room to help you navigate.*

Comparing the normal or expected findings to the "abnormal" findings this evening leads you to conclude that what took place in the home that evening was different than what normally occurs. The current situation represents signs (objective data) of a problem. An investigation with application of other thinking skills is needed prior to arriving at a conclusion about these findings. To further investigate, you collect subjective information (explanation from the children) about what occurred during the evening.

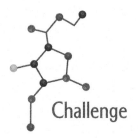

Challenge

Provide an example of how you use the critical thinking skill of "Identifying Signs and Symptoms" in your everyday life.

_____

_____

_____

_____

_____

_____

_____

_____

_____

_____

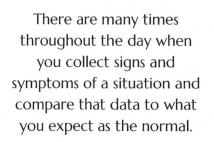

There are many times throughout the day when you collect signs and symptoms of a situation and compare that data to what you expect as the normal.

Example Using "Identifying Signs and Symptoms" in Nursing

You are caring for a patient who is one day post open abdominal surgery for ruptured appendix. To understand what you might expect, prior to visiting your patient you read the textbook explanation of this condition which gives the following information.

Expected Clinical Picture

- *Vital signs within normal limits for patient*

- *Relief of pain with patient controlled analgesia*

- *Abdominal dressing in place, dry and intact*

- *Clear, straw-colored urine in urinary drainage bag*

- *IV solution as ordered and running at prescribed rate*

- *Alert and oriented to person, place, and time, if this was the level of functioning prior to the surgery*

When you visit your patient your assessment reveals:

- *Vital signs are within patient's normal range*

- *The patient rates pain a 3 on a 0 to 10 scale*

- *The dressing is intact but there is an area of fresh blood. The patient states it was not there an hour ago.*

- *The urine in the drainage bag is clear, straw-colored, and about 150 milliliters (emptied one hour ago)*

- *The IV solution and rate are as prescribed*

- *The patient is awake and oriented to person, place, and time*

When you compare and contrast the textbook "normal" findings with your patient assessment data, you find that all seems well with the exception of the fresh blood on the dressing. More investigation with application of other thinking skills is needed to make conclusions based on this finding.

Assessing Systematically and Comprehensively

Definition

Assessing systematically and comprehensively is a thinking skill applied to all areas of nursing practice. For example, when assessing patients, nurses use a systematic method such as a body systems or a head-to-toe approach so no areas are missed.

A systematic and comprehensive approach is also used for data collection during a shift report. Most nurses use a specific format for gathering patient data to ensure all important areas of information are noted.

Example Using "Assessing Systematically and Comprehensively" in Everyday Life

You are shopping for a new car. Because you have experience purchasing a car you realize how salespersons may distract you with features of a car in an effort to sell the vehicle. To prevent becoming distracted by the salesperson you decide you need to list important features you want in the car to avoid being persuaded to buy a car without what you desire because the salesperson focused on other features. Therefore, prior to visiting the first car dealer you realize the importance of identifying what you are looking for in this new car. You develop a list of car features you find important.

To be sure you don't miss any important features you group them into categories. Your list may look something like this:

CAR ASSESSMENT

Performance Features

- *4 cylinder*
- *25 miles to the gallon*
- *Good pick-up when passing another car*

Safety Features

- *Backup camera*
- *Blind spot indicator on side mirrors*
- *Beeper for close contact with an object*

Pleasure/Comfort Features

- *Satellite radio*
- *Heated steering wheel*
- *USB port in the front*
- *Heated seats in both front seats (perhaps in the back if possible)*
- *Smooth ride in the back seat*

When you visit car dealers you find your evaluation of possible cars to purchase is controlled, without distraction from the salesperson. Your assessment is systematic and comprehensive; comprehensive meaning you are not missing any of the important features you want in this vehicle. Awareness of these features and a systematic approach to your assessment yield the most reliable information on which to make a decision and take action.

> Assessing systematically
> and comprehensively is a
> thinking skill applied to all
> areas of nursing practice.

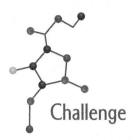

Challenge

Provide an example of how you use the critical thinking skill of "Assessing Systematically and Comprehensively" in your everyday life.

_____

_____

_____

_____

_____

_____

_____

_____

_____

_____

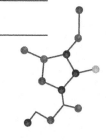

Nurses use a systematic
approach as a form
of mental discipline to
ensure comprehensive
data collection.

Example Using "Assessing Systematically and Comprehensively" in Nursing

Assessing systematically serves the purpose of being comprehensive; that is, when an assessment of any type is performed based on a systematic approach, that approach provides the best chance for a comprehensive assessment. Comprehensive implies a complete assessment that yields all data important to the situation. A systematic approach is used to ensure nothing important is left out of the assessment. Nurses use a systematic approach as a form of mental discipline to ensure comprehensive data collection.

An example of assessing systematically and comprehensively relates to ensuring a safe environment. The nurse assesses the patient and the patient's environment to ensure safety. Some important factors to consider include the following:

SAFETY ASSESSMENT

Patient

- Positioning

- Nonslip socks

- Tubes

- Equipment

- Other factors to consider for this particular patient:

_____

_____

Environment
- Clutter

- Height of the bed

- Call light within reach

- Glove supply

- Needle receptacle

- Other factors for this particular healthcare setting/unit:

_____

_____

There are many important safety factors to consider with each patient and the patient's environment. Using a tool such as this list that organizes all these factors provides a comprehensive safety assessment. Organizing the factors into groups then referencing each of these groups as a way to systematically organize your thinking helps to ensure a comprehensive assessment. Repeated use of this tool helps your thinking become automatic. Revise this list by adding more items as you learn more about nursing.

GATHERING ACCURATE INFORMATION

Definition

Gathering accurate information is fundamental to critical thinking and clinical judgment/clinical reasoning. Data are collected from all sources available to the nurse, but the data must be accurate. The data are then used as the basis for solving problems and making decisions, so it is important that not only the processes used for data collection but the data themselves are accurate. The sources of data must be deemed reliable and the processes used to gather the data must be skillfully performed. To meet this goal, nurses must be confident in their abilities to know what data to collect, how to accurately collect the data, and how to ensure the data are accurate.

Example Using "Gathering Accurate Information" in Everyday Life

As you are shopping for a new car it is important to gather accurate data about the car prior to purchase. To gather accurate data you identify sources of information that are reliable. Sources of information include:

- Manufacturer's website
- Vehicle rating websites
- Acquaintances who own a similar make and model
- If this is a used car, a reliable website that gives the history of the car's accidents

Based on information gleaned from these reliable sources of accurate information you are prepared to visit car dealers. This information is used to balance the information provided by other sources of information that may be less reliable in accuracy such as the sales person who has a personal interest in selling the car.

Another Example Using "Gathering Accurate Information" in Everyday Life

You are driving on the highway. A police officer turns on the flashing lights and pulls you over. The officer states you were clocked driving 15 miles per hour above the posted speed limit. She states she used a speed gun to record your speed. It is the officer's responsibility to ensure the device is functioning properly so the data recorded are accurate.

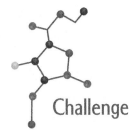

Challenge

Provide an example of how you use the critical thinking skill of "Gathering Accurate Information" in your everyday life.

_____

_____

_____

_____

_____

_____

_____

_____

_____

Nurses must be confident in
their abilities to know what
data to collect,
how to accurately
collect the data,
and how to ensure
the data are accurate.

Example Using "Gathering Accurate Information" in Nursing

Nurses review patient laboratory results that measure various body functions. If a laboratory result is out of range and reaches a critical level, another sample may be collected and compared to the first result to ensure the results are accurate. Reasons for the repeat in testing are to determine if the instrument is functioning correctly or if the process was accurately implemented to yield reliable data.

Another example of ensuring the information nurses collect is accurate is the selection of a blood pressure cuff. The blood pressure cuff is selected based on the size of the patient's arm. The wrong size cuff can yield inaccurate readings.

Another important aspect of gathering accurate data is the source of the information nurses use. As nurses care for patients, they must identify and locate reliable sources of accurate information.

Some of the sources of information include:

- Professional online websites for sources of current information

- Experienced nurses with whom you are working

- Your nursing teacher/preceptor

- Textbooks and other reference materials with a current copyright date

Finally, the nurse assesses the patient's ability to provide an accurate history. If the patient is experiencing confusion or dementia, or is under the influence of a narcotic medication, the patient may not be an accurate source of information. Ensuring the patient is a reliable historian is an important aspect of gathering accurate information.

> Sources of data must be
> deemed reliable and
> the processes used to
> gather the data must be
> skillfully performed.

PREDICTING POTENTIAL COMPLICATIONS

Definition

Potential complications are possible for most patients receiving nursing care. Predicting potential complications is a major responsibility of the nurse and requires critical thinking. Nurses must look at the total patient picture to predict potential complications that may exist for individual patients. Many conditions inherently have potential complications that might occur which is why nurses include measures focused at prevention.

A more extreme way of looking at the thinking skill of predicting potential complications is early recognition of predictable emergencies. If measures are not put into place to prevent potential complications, then an emergency situation is highly probable. If the patient's condition deteriorates and the patient dies, this is considered a failure to rescue situation. It is obvious that failure to rescue is extremely undesirable.

The starting point for predicting potential complications is to know common complications related to a patient's condition. For example, developing a blood clot in the leg from lack of movement due to bed rest or limitations on ambulation. Then consider individual patient differences that may result in additional concerns for that patient. A blood clot in the leg may be caused by bed rest, but further exploration of individual patient differences may raise your level of concern such as the patient smokes and takes birth control pills, both of which contribute to blood clots. A major nursing activity is to ensure preventable complications are indeed prevented.

> Nurses must look at
> the total patient picture
> to predict potential
> complications that
> may exist for
> individual patients.

Example Using "Predicting Potential Complications" in Everyday Life

There are often times in everyday life when you predict potential complications. One example is predicting complications when weather threatens your commute home after work.

> *The weather forecast is for snow during the time you are at work. You predict you may have complications with your commute home if this happens, so you plan to manage any complications that may result. Before you can manage potential complications, you must first think*

ahead to determine what those possible complications might be then prepare yourself should any of the possible complications occur.

In nursing thinking ahead is called clinical forethought. In this example, potential complications may be:

- You are delayed in your car for long periods of time and run out of gas.

- You are delayed so long you miss dinner time and may get very hungry.

- You may need to turn off the car at times to conserve gasoline and the car becomes cold.

- You may need to call for help using your cell phone.

Once you determine the possible complications, you realize you must manage those potential complications should they occur. Managing potential complications is a thinking skill listed under the Interpreting Step. To manage the complications that may occur in this example you do the following:

- Before leaving for work you fill your car's fuel tank with gas.

- You pack cold weather outerwear.

- You take healthy snacks and water.

- You ensure your cellular phone is fully charged.

You continue to monitor the weather during the day. Once the snow begins to fall at an alarmingly fast rate, you alert your supervisor who has the authority to close the business establishment early if needed. By predicting the weather may cause complications related to a safe commute home, you prepared to deal with those complications should they occur. Your goal is to totally prevent complications from occurring or minimize any harmful effects should a complication occur.

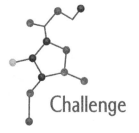

Challenge

Provide an example of how you use the critical thinking skill of "Predicting Potential Complications" in your everyday life.

_____

_____

_____

_____

_____

_____

_____

_____

_____

_____

Your goal is to totally
prevent complications
from occurring or minimize
any harmful effects
should a complication occur.

Example Using "Predicting Potential Complications" in Nursing

Most surgical patients are at risk for potential complications such as atelectasis and pneumonia. Interventions such as deep breathing and coughing exercises, early ambulation, and the use of an incentive spirometer are planned. However, an 18-year-old athlete in excellent physical condition who has undergone a laparoscopic appendectomy is at much less risk for these complications than a 60-year-old obese patient with a history of cigarette smoking who has undergone a colon resection. Therefore, individual factors for these two patients dictate the degree to which the preventive measures are taken. That is, the care the nurse plans to prevent complications after surgery is directly related to the individual patient situation. The 60-year-old patient may need to use the incentive spirometer more frequently than the 18-year-old athlete.

Another example is a patient in your care who has a very slow pulse rate, 38 beats per minute. A potential complication is dizziness. Therefore, you ensure an alarm is in place to alert you if the patient gets out of bed alone because the dizziness may result in a fall causing even more possible complications.

The nurse must engage in **clinical forethought**, thinking ahead to foresee any possible complications for each individual patient. Interventions to prevent complications or to minimize the effects of complications require clinical judgment to ensure the patient is safe while under your care.

> The nurse must engage
> in *clinical forethought,*
> thinking ahead to
> foresee any possible
> complications for each
> individual patient.

Interpreting Step

The thinking skills used in the Noticing Step yield information about the patient or situation. The Interpreting Step requires you to analyze the data to make sense of all the data collected. In the Interpreting Step once you sort through the information collected and analyze the information, you use the data to develop a plan.

The thinking skills and strategies used in this step help answer questions such as:

- What do the data mean?

- How should the data be interpreted for this patient?

- What are the most important data?

- What actions should be planned?

- How should the actions be prioritized?

Therefore, in the Interpreting Step your goal is to:

- Process the information you "noticed"—data collected related to the patient and/or the healthcare environment.

- Analyze that data to arrive at a clear, accurate understanding of the situation.

- Based on your understanding of the situation, determine actions you will take.

The end product of the Interpreting Step is your plan. That is, once all the data have been interpreted and analyzed, and you have a clear, accurate understanding of the situation, you use the information to formulate a plan of care for the patient or plan of action for dealing with an issue within the healthcare environment. When developing your plan of care or plan of action you apply legal, ethical, and professional guidelines to ensure your plan is acceptable. This means you must have knowledge of these guidelines, which is part of your nursing education. In addition, you use the policies and procedures of the healthcare institution to provide specific information about how to carry out nursing care and nursing actions in that agency. You will also need to be cognizant of position descriptions for those with whom you work. For example, if you are working with a nursing assistant, you must be aware of the job description for that position.

Accurate interpretation of the data is critical if you are to provide quality, safe, effective nursing care. There are ten thinking skills and strategies in the Interpreting Step presented in this book:

1. Clustering related information

2. Recognizing inconsistencies

3. Determining important information to collect

4. Distinguishing relevant from irrelevant information

5. Judging how much ambiguity is acceptable

6. Comparing and contrasting

7. Managing potential complications

8. Identifying assumptions

9. Setting priorities

10. Collaborating

CLUSTERING RELATED INFORMATION

Definition

Clustering related information refers to grouping together information with a common theme. This is the process used when formulating nursing diagnoses, when identifying patient problems or concerns, or determining what actions to take. Related signs and symptoms are clustered together along with other pertinent information such as laboratory or diagnostic study results, preexisting conditions, and other information to form the basis for a nursing diagnosis or problem identification.

Clustering related information is foundational to determining the patient's condition, identifying changes in the patient's condition, and determining appropriate responses to prevent patient deterioration. The thinking skill of clustering related information also pertains to solving workplace issues and problems. Identification of information that demonstrates a cause of a workplace issue helps direct the nurse to possible solutions.

Example Using "Clustering Related Information" in Everyday Life

When organizing a large family gathering, the event planner decided to look at the weather forecast to consider holding the event outside. The weather forecast for the day was:

- Sunny conditions

- Temperature of 80 degrees

- Dew point of 72 degrees

- Winds 20 miles per hour with guests up to 35 miles per hour

- UV index: 1 (low)

- Cloud cover: 25%

- Visibility: 10 miles

With these weather details revealing a sunny, clear, warm day, the planner decided to hold the event outside. The planner ordered a tent with tables and chairs for eating the meal, large tables to hold supplies, and lawn game equipment. Over 50 people were invited to the event.

The event was held and proved to be a disaster. The planner did not cluster all related information prior to making decisions. Data the planner did not consider when reviewing the weather forecast were two important elements: dew point and wind. The dew point that day was 72 degrees which means the air was so saturated with moisture attendees were extremely uncomfortable. The winds were sustained at 20 miles an hour with gusts up to 35 miles an hour at times throughout the afternoon. The tent was blown over and everything on the tables that was not weighted down was blown away. It was a very unpleasant event. The planner failed to cluster all the related information prior to making the decision about the event. When clustering related information, all information pertinent to a situation must be collected, but also must be considered as a whole prior to making a decision.

A person's ability to think critically determines if the person is able to cluster the pertinent data for a given situation. In this situation pertinent information included the chance of rain, wind velocity, dew point for comfort when outdoors, and temperature. This same information can be used to make other decisions about the same event. For example, if the person is deciding to take an umbrella on the walk to the event, only two pieces of information are necessary, chance of precipitation and wind velocity. All the information is available, but the individual making the decision must select and cluster the information pertinent to the decision that is being made.

All pertinent data are clustered together and considered as a whole prior to making a decision. The event planner did not cluster all important information prior to making the decision to hold the event outside and this resulted in negative consequences. In this situation, the event planner only chose two pieces of information to cluster to make a decision. Although the event planner was aware of all the data, other important pieces of information were not clustered together with a decision made based on how all those pieces related to each other.

Nurses must use this same thinking skill to first determine what information is important to collect then determine which data to cluster to see the "bigger picture" for that particular patient. This is clinical reasoning that takes place to identify a patient problem, issue, or concern. This is the nursing diagnosis or problem identification piece of the nursing process. The nursing diagnosis may be stated in formal nursing diagnosis terminology or may be stated as a patient problem. Whether a nursing diagnosis or patient problem verbiage is used depends on the healthcare system.

> Nurses must use this same thinking skill to first determine what information is important to collect then determine which data to cluster to see the "bigger picture" for that particular patient.

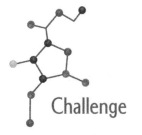

Challenge

Provide an example of how you use the critical thinking skill of "Clustering Related Information" in your everyday life.

_____

_____

_____

_____

_____

_____

_____

_____

_____

_____

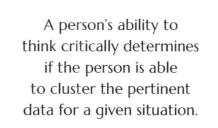

A person's ability to
think critically determines
if the person is able
to cluster the pertinent
data for a given situation.

Example Using "Clustering Related Information" in Nursing

The patient care plan includes a reminder to call the primary healthcare provider if the patient's temperature is above 102 degrees Fahrenheit. The nursing assistant reports a temperature of 103 degrees. Before calling the physician the nurse knows other information is important to gather that relates to an elevated temperature, such as:

- *White blood cell count from the morning's complete blood count (CBC) report*

- *Previous temperatures and how this 103 degree reading compares; this is known as looking at the "trend"*

- *Blood pressure, heart rate, and respiratory rate that may indicate further problems*

- *Medications previously administered such as antibiotics and antipyretic agents*

Clustering this information related to the elevated temperature reading is needed to provide a complete picture when reporting to the primary healthcare provider. Competency in using the thinking skill of clustering related information depends on the nurse's ability to identify information related to the situation at hand.

RECOGNIZING INCONSISTENCIES

Definition

The beginning point of the nursing process is assessment. While assessing, both subjective and objective data are collected. In reviewing the data, nurses use the thinking skill of recognizing inconsistencies among all the subjective and the objective data that may indicate additional problems that are not readily apparent. Consider subjective data that indicate one issue but the objective data do not support the presence of that issue. For example, the patient states he feels he is "burning up" and must have a high fever. The nurse takes the patient's temperature which is 99.0 degrees Fahrenheit. These two pieces of information are inconsistent.

This is also true when gathering information about the healthcare environment. For example, a nursing assistant is responsible for taking and recording vital signs for ten patients. Within 20 minutes after starting this task he states he has taken all the patients' vital signs and they are all recorded. The nurse would suspect a possible inconsistency with that information because the amount of time in which the vital signs were taken and recorded is not consistent with the time expected to complete the task.

Example Using "Recognizing Inconsistencies" in Everyday Life

Upon rising in the morning it is common for people to exercise. A runner looks at her phone to determine the weather over the next hour to determine if she should run outside or use the treadmill in her basement. The weather application reports rain with a chance of thunderstorms currently and for the next two hours. A look outside shows sunny skies with broken clouds. The information from these two sources is inconsistent. The runner is now faced with the decision about which is correct. Is the application on the phone wrong and the weather will be dry for a 45 minute run? Or, in the next 45 minutes will rain move in and she will be outside when the rain, or worse yet, a thunderstorm arrives?

This situation is an example of collecting data and identifying inconsistencies. To deal with the issue and make a decision requires using other thinking skills such as determining the accuracy of the data or perhaps predicting and managing potential complications should she decide to run outside and it begins to storm.

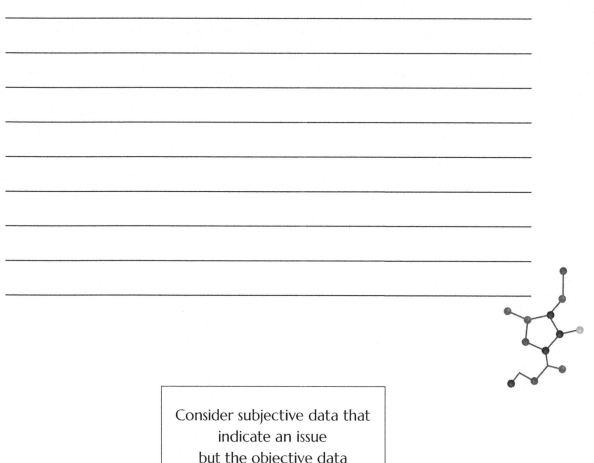

Challenge

Provide an example of how you use the critical thinking skill of "Recognizing Inconsistencies" in your everyday life.

_____

_____

_____

_____

_____

_____

_____

_____

_____

Consider subjective data that
indicate an issue
but the objective data
do not support the
presence of that issue.

Example Using "Recognizing Inconsistencies" in Nursing

In addition to the above example about the nursing assistant taking vital signs, here is another example when a nurse may need to use the thinking skill of recognizing inconsistencies.

> *When completing an admission database on a 23-year-old female patient, the nurse notes the patient is 5 feet 8 inches tall, thin, pale, and weighs 103 pounds. The patient denies a history of psychological problems, eating disorders, or gastrointestinal pathology. She states she is very busy with her career and school, but is able to eat 3 complete meals a day. She also eats an occasional between-meal snack. She states she is fortunate she is physically active because that helps control her body weight. Blood studies revealed a hemoglobin of 9.8g/dL (normal is 13.5 to 17.5 g/dL) and a total serum protein of 4.8 g/dL (normal is 6.3-7.9 g/dL). The subjective and objective information reveal inconsistencies that might indicate a possible eating disorder.*

DETERMINING IMPORTANT INFORMATION TO COLLECT

Definition

Nurses face a myriad of information to sort through for every patient. This information may change often throughout the course of a day. Therefore, nurses must be able to determine what information to collect that is important to the care of the patient that day. Then, throughout the day the nurse must determine what information is important to collect to identify any changes in the patient's condition. Once important data are collected, the nurse can determine what data are actually relevant then act on that data.

Example Using "Determining Important Information to Collect" in Everyday Life

> *You are at the Newark, New Jersey airport scheduled on a direct, nonstop flight to the Los Angeles Airport (LAX). Your plane is delayed an hour, then another hour. Finally the airline announces the flight has been canceled. You immediately start to collect important information to try to arrive in Los Angeles today. You collect information about:*
>
> - Direct flights on your scheduled airline going to Los Angeles
>
> - Connecting flights on your scheduled airline going to Los Angeles
>
> - Flights on your scheduled airline going to other Los Angeles airports such as the John Wayne airport or the Ontario airport
>
> - Flights going to Los Angeles or a nearby airport on another airline

You have approximately 10 flights that are a possibility for you to select to meet your goal of arriving in Los Angeles this evening. Once you have all this important information you will use the next thinking step (distinguishing relevant from irrelevant information) to further analyze the data.

Challenge

Provide an example of how you use the critical thinking skill of "Determining Important Information to Collect" in your everyday life.

_____

_____

_____

_____

_____

_____

_____

_____

_____

Nurses must be able to
determine what information
to collect that is important
to the care of the
patient that day.

Example Using "Determining Important Information to Collect" in Nursing

The nurse is caring for a patient who is two days post abdominal surgery. The patient has a history of diabetes mellitus, hypertension, frequent urinary tract infections, and coronary artery disease. When visiting the patient at 8:30 AM the patient states she is feeling a little dizzy and is somewhat confused in her thinking. The nurse decides to collect information that is important related to this patient's report of her current condition. Taking into consideration the patient's surgery and pre-existing conditions, the nurse decides to check the patient's blood sugar, blood pressure, and level of pain at the surgical site as well as any chest discomfort. The nurse also observes the urine in the urinary drainage bag.

There are many other assessments the nurse might make for this patient relative to her overall condition, but the nurse must decide specific information that is important to the patient's new report of dizziness and slight confusion considering her current postoperative status as well as her past medical history. Once the data are collected the nurse must determine which of those data are relevant. Distinguishing relevant from irrelevant information for this situation is discussed with the next thinking skill.

Distinguishing Relevant from Irrelevant Information

Definition

The thinking skill of distinguishing relevant from irrelevant information refers to the nurse deciding which information is pertinent or connects with the matter at hand. All information about a patient may be important for the patient's overall care, but the nurse must sort out which information is relevant to a particular problem or situation currently under consideration.

Example Using "Distinguishing Relevant from Irrelevant Information" in Everyday Life

Remember the situation from the previous thinking skill: determining important information to collect? It went like this:

You are at the Newark, New Jersey airport scheduled on a direct, nonstop flight to the Los Angeles Airport (LAX). Your plane is delayed an hour, then another hour. Finally the airline announces the flight has been canceled. You immediately start to collect important information to try to arrive in Los Angeles today. You collect information about:

- Direct flights on your scheduled airline going to Los Angeles

- Connecting flights on your scheduled airline going to Los Angeles

- Flights on your scheduled airline going to other Los Angeles airports such as the John Wayne airport or the Ontario airport

- Flights going to Los Angeles or nearby airport on another airline

You have approximately 10 flights that are a possibility for you to select to meet your goal of arriving in Los Angeles this evening.

Now that you have collected all that information you must distinguish between the relevant and irrelevant information. You'll need to determine considerations for this thinking task. Considerations include:

- What is the terminal and gate each of the 10 flights is leaving from? Is that terminal and gate in close proximity to you?

- How much time is there before each of the 10 flights leave? Do you have time to get from where you are currently to the departing gate to make that flight?

- How many other people are on the stand-by list who are trying to also get on each of those flights?

- For flights arriving at another Los Angeles area airport, will you have ground transportation from that airport to your home?

- If you request the airline to put you on a flight with another airline, will you have to pay a fee?

Once you determine which flights are actually feasible, you have distinguished which information is relevant for your solution and which is not relevant. You have determined only five flights will actually work for you. Now you might prioritize those flights prior to talking with an airline agent.

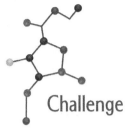

Challenge

Provide an example of how you use the critical thinking skill of "Distinguishing Relevant from Irrelevant Information" in your everyday life.

_____

_____

_____

_____

_____

_____

_____

_____

_____

_____

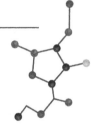

Nurses face a myriad of
information to sort
through for every patient.
This information may change
often throughout the
course of a day.

Example Using "Distinguishing Relevant from Irrelevant Information" in Nursing

Remember the situation from the previous thinking skill: determining important information to collect? It went like this:

> *The nurse is caring for a patient who is two days post abdominal surgery. The patient has a history of diabetes mellitus, hypertension, frequent urinary tract infection, and coronary artery disease. When visiting the patient at 8:30 AM the patient states she is feeling little dizzy and is somewhat confused in her thinking. The nurse decides to collect information that is important related to this patient's report of her current condition. The nurse decides to check the patient's blood sugar, blood pressure, and level of pain at the surgical site as well as any chest discomfort. The nurse also observes the urine in the urinary drainage bag. There are many other assessments the nurse might make for this patient relative to her overall condition, but the nurse must decide specific information that is important to this current change in the patient's condition of dizziness and slight confusion. Once the data are collected the nurse must determine which of those data are relevant.*

> *The nurse has collected the important data for the patient's report of dizziness and slight confusion. The results are as follows:*

> - Blood sugar of 56 (low)
>
> - Blood pressure of 130/90 (within patient's normal)
>
> - Level of pain at the surgical site: 4 on a 0 to 10 scale (pain is moderately controlled)
>
> - Denies chest discomfort (no indication of a cardiac event)
>
> - Urine is clear and amber color (no indication of a urinary tract infection on visual inspection)

The nurse collected important information that was specific for this patient's current issue based on the patient's history and current postoperative status. The nurse did not immediately make a decision about what was causing the symptoms, but collected important information specific for this patient. The nurse then analyzes the data collected to determine which data are relevant and might be contributing to the patient's report of dizziness and slight confusion. Analysis of the information leads the nurse to take action about the low blood sugar. Using these thinking skills results in an accurate determination about the source of the patient's symptoms that are then addressed with a targeted, effective intervention.

Here is another example:

> *The nurse is caring for a patient four hours after a cardiac cauterization. When the nurse ambulates the patient the site begins to bleed profusely. The nurse hurriedly returns the patient to the bed, applies pressure on the bleeding site, and asks the nursing assistant to take a set of vital signs. The nursing assistant replies she would have to go to the nurses' station for a thermometer. The nurse quickly restates his request with, "Take a blood pressure and a pulse, please."*

In this situation when the nursing assistant heard "a set of vital signs," she was unable to distinguish which vital signs were relevant and which were not. It was important for the nurse to intervene and ask the nursing assistant to take only the relevant vital signs to expedite the collection of data about the patient's current status and to establish a baseline should the patient's condition worsen. The thinking skill of distinguishing relevant from irrelevant information was crucial in this situation.

JUDGING HOW MUCH AMBIGUITY IS ACCEPTABLE

Definition

Ambiguity refers to being unclear, uncertain, or vague. Life has many rules that are used to provide order in a society or guidelines for approaching a problem. However, there are times when a rule cannot be applied exactly as written. Ambiguity occurs when factors relating to a situation make applying the rule somewhat grey. That is, the rule is not always strictly applied because of specific circumstances of a given situation. Many situations appear similar on the surface but actually differ when all factors about that situation are carefully considered. Therefore, the approach to dealing with that situation requires a close look and analysis.

When ambiguity is present in a situation, application of a rule may require some "wiggle room." That is, the situation may require going outside the limits of the rule which is typically acceptable based on the details of the situation. When a rule is not strictly applied, it is important to use the facts about the situation to justify modification of the rule for that situation. It is this phenomenon that explains the commonly held belief that nursing is not black or white but gray. Gray means that rather than strict application of a rule or guideline, application "depends" on the situation.

Example Using "Judging How Much Ambiguity is Acceptable" in Everyday Life

> *When driving a car and merging onto an expressway, a rule is considered. That rule is the speed limit, with the maximum and minimum limits posted. However, before deciding how much "wiggle room" there is when considering the actual rate of speed that will be driven, the driver collects data.*

That data may include:

- Amount of traffic

- Weather conditions

- Visibility

- Condition of the road

- Location of police officers

- Number of traffic violations the driver has

After very quickly considering all the data, the driver makes a decision about what speed **above** the posted limit can be safely driven. Or, if the data reveal issues with weather or road conditions, how much **slower** to drive than the posted minimum.

> Ambiguity occurs when factors relating to a situation make applying the rule somewhat grey.
> That is, the rule is not always strictly applied because of specific circumstances of a given situation.

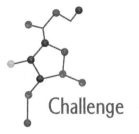

Challenge

Provide an example of how you use the critical thinking skill of "Judging How Much Ambiguity is Acceptable" in your everyday life.

_____

_____

_____

_____

_____

_____

_____

_____

_____

_____

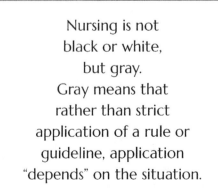

Nursing is not
black or white,
but gray.
Gray means that
rather than strict
application of a rule or
guideline, application
"depends" on the situation.

Example Using "Judging How Much Ambiguity is Acceptable" in Nursing

In the beginning nursing course students learn the psychomotor skill of taking vital signs. They learn the "within normal limits" rules of vital signs. It is critical for nurses to decide how much ambiguity can be tolerated for an individual patient around the "within normal limits" of vital signs. Using this skill the situation is considered and a rule applied, not in a strict sense, but in a "how much wiggle room" can be tolerated when applying the rule. For example:

> *The nursing assistant reports to the nurse that patient #1's blood pressure is 100/60 and patient #2's blood pressure is 105/60. Based on the information the nurse obtained in the shift report, the nurse knows that he must immediately assess patient #2 (BP of 105/60), but patient's #1 (BP of 100/60) can wait.*

How can this be? The nurse made this decision by considering other information related to the condition of each patient. The nurse looked at the context of each patient. Patient #1's blood pressure is normal for that patient. Patient #2 is a newly admitted trauma victim under observation for internal injuries. Her blood pressure readings have not been lower than 130/85. With the blood pressure now 105/60, the nurse needs to immediately visit patient #2 to further assess the situation.

COMPARING AND CONTRASTING

Definition

The thinking skill of comparing and contrasting looks at two or more situations that are similar by some common characteristic. With further study, differences between the two situations emerge. Many situations appear similar on the surface but actually differ when all factors are carefully considered. These differences may not be readily apparent for those unfamiliar with the type of situations under consideration. As one becomes more familiar and has experience working with similar situations, small variances or differences become readily apparent. Small differences or variances are also known as nuances. Nuances are very slight differences or variations that can greatly affect decisions that are made.

Example Using "Comparing and Contrasting" in Everyday Life

Some common situations in which you might use comparing and contrasting include:

- Comparing your weight to a chart

- Comparing two or more toddlers in their ability to talk or perform a motor skill

- Comparing the length of one side of your hair to the other during a haircut to ensure they are even

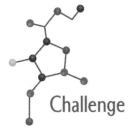

Challenge

Provide an example of how you use the critical thinking skill of "Comparing and Contrasting" in your everyday life.

_____

_____

_____

_____

_____

_____

_____

_____

_____

Many situations
appear similar on the
surface but actually
differ when all factors
are carefully considered.

Example Using "Comparing and Contrasting" in Nursing

Engaging in comparing and contrasting helps nurses recognize differences and similarities among patients or situations. These differences may be evident or they may be very subtle. Subtle differences are called nuances. These differences or nuances can make a patient or situation unique.

The more experience comparing and contrasting patients and situations, the more individualized patient care becomes. For example:

> *The nurse is caring for two patients who are both one day postoperative with the same surgery. The nurse must decide how far to ambulate each patient. The nurse decides to ambulate one patient around the entire unit but decides to ambulate the second patient only to the door of the patient's room then back to the chair. Although both patients had the same surgery and are both in postop day 1, the small differences, or nuances, between the two patients led the nurse to safely determine the acceptable distance for each patient.*

Comparing and contrasting can also be applied to one patient. Remember, any time a patient has two of "something", such as two arms, always compare the one being investigated with the other that appears to be normal. For example, the nurse looks at the patient's IV site. It appears a little swollen. The nurse is unsure if this is the normal size of the patient's arm or if it is a result of an infiltration of the IV fluid into the tissues rather than the vein. The nurse then compares the arm with the IV to the arm without an IV for the purpose of making the determination.

MANAGING POTENTIAL COMPLICATIONS

Definition

Under the Noticing Step of the Clinical Judgment Model, you learned about predicting potential complications. In the Interpreting Step it is important to determine how you can best manage the potential complications that were identified.

Example Using "Managing Potential Complications" in Everyday Life

A common complication in everyday life is a problem with traffic.

> *You are driving to work and signs begin to appear that alert you to construction ahead. Traffic is starting to slow. You look at the GPS which notes slowed then stopped traffic for the next 5 miles. As you consider this information you predict there is a problem with backed up traffic. You consider the complications that may result if you do not arrive at your destination on time. The complications are:*

- *Late for work*

- *Run out of gas*

To manage complications you begin to consider interventions to implement. These interventions might include:

- Take the next exit which is in 1 mile; the GPS indicates the traffic on the alternate route is slow but not stopped

- Stay on the route and notify employer of a likely late arrival

- Locate nearest gas station on the highway

You must manage the potential complications resulting from change in your normal drive to work.

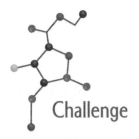

Challenge

Provide an example of how you use the critical thinking skill of "Managing Potential Complications" in your everyday life.

_____

_____

_____

_____

_____

_____

_____

_____

_____

The nurse prepares for managing potential complications by using the thinking skill during the Noticing Step of predicting potential complications, then in the Interpreting Step addressing how to manage the identified potential complications.

Example Using "Managing Potential Complications" in Nursing

Some patients in the acute care setting receive narcotics to control pain. Administration of the narcotic is often via a system where the patient self-administers the narcotic by pushing a button to release intravenous medication. A potential complication in this case is a decreasing respiratory rate. The nurse knows to closely monitor the patient's respiratory rate. However, should the respiratory rate drop too low, perhaps below 12 breaths per minute, the nurse must know how to manage that complication. Planning what to do prior to the event actually happening is extremely important and is known as clinical forethought. The nurse prepares for managing potential complications by using the thinking skill during the Noticing Step of predicting potential complications, then in the Interpreting Step addressing how to manage the identified potential complications. Although presented in this book as clearly two steps in the thinking process, the nurse automatically carries out these two steps together as one.

IDENTIFYING ASSUMPTIONS

Definition

Everyone's perception of the world is shaped by life experiences. It is critical that each nurse considers personal biases that are brought to the practice setting. Nurses do not intentionally use negative assumptions in a patient situation. However, remember, a patient may be a prisoner who committed a murder or a sex offense. Some health issues such as alcoholism or drug addiction are processed in many ways by the public. These circumstances may affect the nurse's opinion of the patient. Other areas of life such as a patient's religion, race, or sexual orientation may be different from that of the nurse. Nurses may not have much experience with some of these aspects of a patient's life or lifestyle and may make assumptions that interfere with quality care.

It is important for nurses to identify any assumptions they have about a patient and recognize there is no place for personal opinions and biases. Nurses must recognize that the rights of patients come before the beliefs of the nurse. Nurses are non-judgmental. Identifying your own assumptions is critical for you to be able to seek the truth about the situation even if what you find is contrary to your own lifestyle and beliefs. Your ability to identify assumptions is rooted in being receptive to other views and sensitive to your own biases (Rubenfeld & Scheffer, 2015). Not being able to sort through assumptions and biases that may influence your thinking can result in unequal or unfair treatment of patients and others with whom you work.

Example Using "Identifying Assumptions" in Everyday Life

Assumptions people hold are not always obvious. Some not so obvious assumptions are those commonly held about the elderly. Examples include assuming all elderly people over the age of 70 are "slow" in their thinking; or that most people over the age of 80 live in nursing homes. It is important to recognize any possible assumptions held that are without basis in fact. Nursing care is based on facts not assumptions.

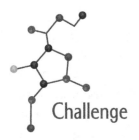

Challenge

Provide an example of how you use the critical thinking skill of "Identifying Assumptions" in your everyday life.

_____

_____

_____

_____

_____

_____

_____

_____

_____

It is important for nurses
to identify any assumptions
they have about a patient
and recognize there is no
place for personal
opinions and biases.

Example Using "Identifying Assumptions" in Nursing

There are many situations in nursing that trigger an emotional response for the nurse. Part of the nurse's assessment is to ask the patient if he/she feels safe at home. The answer may indicate possible domestic abuse. Further discussion with the patient may reveal domestic abuse has been an issue for many years for that patient. An assumption some hold is, if the person is being abused, and especially for a long time, why didn't the person just leave? It is a commonly held belief that if the person doesn't leave, he/she has accepted the abusive relationship. This often leads to a lack of empathy from the nurse.

Once the nurse is educated in domestic abuse it becomes very apparent why the victim does not leave. At that point the false assumption that anyone being abused has the option to "just leave" is often dispelled. However, prior to enlightenment on the subject of domestic abuse it is imperative nurses monitor their own beliefs and not let false assumptions interfere with quality care.

SETTING PRIORITIES

Definition

Setting priorities is a thinking skill constantly used by nurses in all healthcare environments. Prioritizing can be a simple task or a complex task that involves using many other thinking skills and strategies. Nursing examples include:

- Caring for a group of patients and deciding which patients to see first, second, etc.

- For each individual patient determining which assessments and interventions are most important and must be carried out first.

In some settings, protocols are in place to help a nurse prioritize. For example, triage nurses in the emergency department (ED) typically follow a procedure in which patients presenting with chest pain or other cardiac symptoms take priority. For other patients ED nurses use their established knowledge base and experience to determine which patients must be seen first.

Example Using "Setting Priorities" in Everyday Life

Setting priorities is a very common critical thinking skill used in everyday life. You may set and reset priorities many times throughout the day. One example is:

> *You forget to set your alarm and you over sleep. You eventually wake up but you wake up ½ hour late. You typically need 1 1/2 hours to get ready for work in the morning. Since you are*

½ hour late, you must now revise your normal routine. Some of the routine tasks may not get done. How do you reset your priorities with the reduced amount of time? On a typical morning after you wake up you:

- *Exercise*

- *Shower*

- *Dress*

- *Eat breakfast*

- *Gather all your materials for work*

- *Walk the dog*

You must reprioritize this list and perhaps even change the items on the list. You ask yourself:

- What tasks must be done?

- What tasks can be left undone?

- What are the consequences if a task is left undone?

You then prioritize what you can do in an hour rather than the typical 1 1/2 hours you need to get ready for work.

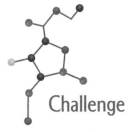

Challenge

Provide an example of how you use the critical thinking skill of "Setting Priorities" in your everyday life.

_____

_____

_____

_____

_____

_____

_____

_____

_____

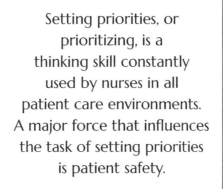

Setting priorities, or
prioritizing, is a
thinking skill constantly
used by nurses in all
patient care environments.
A major force that influences
the task of setting priorities
is patient safety.

Example Using "Setting Priorities" in Nursing

Setting priorities, or prioritizing, is a thinking skill constantly used by nurses in all patient care environments. For example:

> *The nurse is caring for five patients and is working with one nursing assistant. After receiving report from the nurse on the previous shift, the nurse must prioritize what he/she will do.*

A major force that influences the task of setting priorities is patient safety. To ensure all five patients are safe, the nurse determines the order in which to visit each patient. Information from the shift report guides the nurse's thinking about this first task. Some factors to consider include:

- The stability of each patient's condition. That is, are any of the patients' conditions changing frequently and do these patients need close monitoring?

- Are any patients at risk for injury due to conditions such as confusion or dizziness?

- Are any patients requesting, or are due for, pain medication?

- Do any patients have critical medications to be administered immediately such as a cardiac medication or insulin?

These are examples of factors nurses consider when determining how to prioritize their work. Every environment is different thus the factors to consider when prioritizing vary depending on the patient population and healthcare setting.

COLLABORATING WITH OTHER HEALTHCARE TEAM MEMBERS

Definition

The resolution to a problem or approach to care seldom happens while working alone; many people can be involved. In soliciting information and suggestions from others, new perspectives on a problem are realized. Various approaches and solutions may be considered.

Healthcare settings are complex environments requiring the input and cooperation of many members working as a team. Team members engage in critical thinking processes when they examine delivery of care, noting compliance with standards of care and adherence to accepted protocols. This team approach, with all members collaborating and working together, strengthens patient care and fosters positive outcomes.

There are some considerations to make prior to initiating a conversation with another healthcare team member. First, you need to think through the problem and determine the reason for collaborating. In doing so, organize your thoughts and have a system for communicating your concerns, including all pertinent data. Healthcare facilities have adopted a system called ISBAR with many adaptations and modifications from this basic form. The purpose of using the ISBAR format is to ensure a systematic process for complete and accurate exchange of information.

Second, know that conflict may occur. Conflict cannot be avoided. Nurses often work in a rapidly paced environment, full of urgency and serious consequences if errors are made. In this type of environment, conflict is inevitable. Nurses in all areas of patient care must be able to maintain calm, avoid conflict, and if conflict should occur, handle it in a constructive manner. These characteristics serve to promote an atmosphere that is optimal for successful and positive collaboration among the members of the healthcare team.

Example Using "Collaborating with Other Group Members"

Humans are social beings and enjoy being a member of a group. As a member of a group there is much collaboration that occurs when that group is called upon to plan an event, resolve an issue, or make a decision about implementing something new. One group member's idea or perspective about the issue is just that: the idea or perspective of one person. It takes collaboration with other members of the group to ensure all pertinent information is collected, to make a decision that is fair and just to all, and to ensure various perspectives are heard and considered. Examples of such groups include a religious group, sports team, or homeowners association. When you are part of a team, you work within that team.

> This team approach,
> with all members
> collaborating and working
> together, strengthens
> patient care and fosters
> positive outcomes.

Challenge

Provide an example of how you use the critical thinking skill of "Collaborating with Others" in your everyday life.

_____

_____

_____

_____

_____

_____

_____

_____

_____

It takes collaboration with other members of the group to ensure all pertinent information is collected, to make a decision that is fair and just to all, and to ensure various perspectives are heard and considered.

Example Using "Collaborating with Other Healthcare Team Members" in Nursing

A nurse is volunteering in a free clinic. The nurse normally works on a medical unit in the local hospital. The nurse is listening to heart sounds of a 55-year-old patient. An extra sound is heard. The nurse is unsure if this is a problem. The patient states he has no knowledge of any heart problem and no one has ever mentioned an extra sound when listening to his heart. The nurse can decide to take no action since the patient has no other signs or symptoms of disease and has no history of a cardiac problem; or, the nurse can choose to collaborate with another healthcare provider. The nurse reports the finding to the nurse practitioner (NP) who operates the clinic. The NP listens to the patient's heart and decides the finding needs a workup. She contacted the physician to order further diagnostic testing. An echocardiogram is ordered.

As a member of the healthcare team the volunteer nurse recognized a possible problem then collaborated with the NP. It is important to note the nurse's lack of expertise in listening to heart sounds did not interfere with collaborating with others. The nurse readily shared with the NP her lack of knowledge and experience with identifying a cardiac problem based on the auscultation of the patient's heart. This nurse did not hesitate to seek help because an aspect of being a professional is to know what you know and what you don't know and seek assistance as needed.

Responding Step

As discussed earlier, the meaning of the data you collected in the second step (Interpreting Step) guides how you will respond to the situation. The second step yielded a patient care plan guiding continuous care of the patient or an intervention to carry out immediately. Or, the Interpreting Step may have resulted in an action plan about a problem in the healthcare setting. The determinations made in the Interpreting Step are important for deciding how and to what degree you will respond.

After planning actions to take, but prior to implementing the actions in the Responding Step, always think ahead and consider what you expect to happen when you implement your plan. Think about what you intend to go right and what could go wrong. Always have a plan for what to do should something go wrong. This is extremely important. For example, you plan to ambulate a patient. The patient is obese, had major surgery the day before, and has received narcotic pain medications. This is the first time ambulating this patient. What might go wrong? Perhaps the patient becomes dizzy and, due to her weight, you may need help dealing with the situation. Perhaps planning for someone else to be at your side until you are sure the patient is safe would be a good strategy. Clinical forethought—thinking ahead about what might happen in a clinical situation—is very important during the Responding Step.

There are three thinking skills and strategies used during the Responding Step of clinical judgment presented in this book:

- Delegating
- Communicating
- Teaching others

DELEGATING

Definition

Delegating means you transfer the responsibility for performing a task to an individual who has been deemed competent to perform that task. The act of delegating involves many components. The delegator must ensure the task is something that can be delegated. For example, an adult cannot delegate the task of driving to the store to a teenager who does not yet have a driver's license. The person delegated to perform the task must have knowledge about and able to perform the task at hand. The person who is delegating must be assured the person is capable of performing the task. The person delegating must provide clear communication about what is being delegated then ensure appropriate supervision of the task as needed. Of course, no task can always be delegated. Circumstances about a particular situation can result in not delegating a task which might otherwise be delegated. To return to the driving example, an adult may delegate to a newly licensed 16-year-old driver to drive alone to the store five blocks away. However, the task of driving alone in heavy traffic on a busy expressway would not be delegated to the same driver. The task of driving can be delegated to the newly licensed driver, but the adult may make a final decision about a specific driving task depending on factors that affect that situation. Delegating a particular task (in this case driving) is not an absolute but is relative depending on the circumstances of the situation.

Delegating requires nurses to engage in assessing, planning, assigning, supervising, and evaluating. Each of these roles requires a high degree of critical thinking and decision making. When engaged in delegation activities, nurses are accountable that the delegation process is accurately and responsibility carried out in all patient care situations. Prior to delegating a task the nurse must be familiar with the job description of the person to whom the nurse is delegating.

Example Using "Delegating" in Everyday Life

A family is a group of people. Within that group each family member has a role which often includes responsibilities. For example:

> Dad may have the responsibility of grocery shopping, mom may have the responsibility of preparing meals, and the children all have chores or tasks they must perform. If someone in the family is unable to perform their designated task, someone else is asked to do so.

Delegation is the act of assigning that task to another person. For example, mom is unable to prepare the meal on Monday evening. The task is delegated to their 15-year-old daughter. However, prior to assigning to the daughter the task of cooking the meal, the mother uses the delegation process. This process includes deciding who is best prepared to perform the task, if that person has the skill level to make the planned meal, and if the person is available to perform that task. Once these decisions are made, the task can be safely delegated. However, thinking ahead about what can go wrong, the mom ensured the dad is home to help should a problem occur.

> Delegating requires nurses to engage in assessing, planning, assigning, supervising, and evaluating. Each of these roles requires a high degree of critical thinking and decision making.

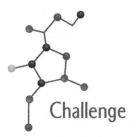

Challenge

Provide an example of how you use the critical thinking skill of "Delegating" in your everyday life.

_____

_____

_____

_____

_____

_____

_____

_____

_____

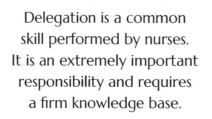

Delegation is a common
skill performed by nurses.
It is an extremely important
responsibility and requires
a firm knowledge base.

Example Using "Delegating" in Nursing

Delegation is a common skill performed by nurses. It is an extremely important responsibility and requires a firm knowledge base. There are important elements to consider, one of which is the state nurse practice act. The nurse practice act in many states indicates which nurses (RNs or LPN/LVNs) are able to delegate nursing tasks to another level of nursing personnel. Another element is the agency's job descriptions. The job description for each of the roles: RN, LPN/LVN, nursing assistant, and other unlicensed assistive personnel indicates that position's responsibilities and what tasks each is permitted to perform. These are important factors to consider when delegating a nursing task.

COMMUNICATING

Definition

Communicating effectively is a highly complex process. Many factors influence communication. Examples of these factors include environment, territoriality, values, personal space, attitudes, and time. The nurse must be aware of these and other factors and not let them block effective communication. It is difficult to carry out effective critical thinking when communication is breaking down.

The principles of therapeutic communication when interacting with patients, as well as guidelines for positive interpersonal communication when interacting with other healthcare providers, are all part of the knowledge base necessary for using the thinking skill of communicating.

Example Using "Communicating" in Everyday Life

People are very social beings and readily communicate with others. Communication is primarily verbal as a child with written and electronic communications included as the person grows and matures.

Communicating clearly is often a difficult skill to master. Clear communication with a toddler and child requires different skills than clear communication with an adult. There are also various types of communication depending on relationships such as social and professional communication. There is also communication with a specific goal such as registering a complaint with a company or inviting others to a party. Any type of communication requires focus and clarity for the communication to be effective.

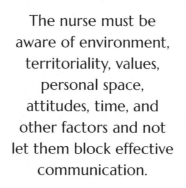

Challenge

Provide an example of how you use the critical thinking skill of "Communicating" in your everyday life.

_____

_____

_____

_____

_____

_____

_____

_____

_____

The nurse must be aware of environment, territoriality, values, personal space, attitudes, time, and other factors and not let them block effective communication.

Example Using "Communicating" in Nursing

Nurses engage in constant communication throughout their daily practice. They communicate with patients, other nursing staff, and other interprofessional healthcare providers. Communicating in nursing is different from communicating in a social setting. Nurses use therapeutic communication techniques and are aware of communication techniques that are not therapeutic. Communication has a goal and purpose. Nurses focus their communication on the **goal of providing quality patient care for the purpose of improving patient outcomes**. In so doing nurses must be very skilled in providing clear, complete communication.

Poor communication between healthcare providers is identified as an issue which can result in poor patient outcomes. To ensure communication among all professionals is clear and concise but complete, most healthcare agencies use a system such as the ISBAR system. The ISBAR mnemonic stands for Identify, Situation, Background, Assessment, and Recommendation. It is a format for communicating in environments that pose a high risk for error from poor communication. Clinical reasoning skills are used to determine what information to include in each of the 5 parts of the ISBAR tool.

TEACHING OTHERS

Definition

In all aspects of life, teaching empowers others. This is true in nursing; nurses empower patients through teaching. Teaching can occur informally any time a nurse interacts with a patient. Teaching is also formalized through the written plan of care. One example of formalized teaching is discharge teaching, which typically addresses specific areas such as medications, diet, activity restrictions, and follow-up visits. Another example of formalized teaching is diabetic teaching, which often involves written guidelines with a checklist to ensure all areas are covered.

Critical thinking skills are used when teaching. Nurses consider all factors, looking at the complete patient situation, to determine what to include in the teaching plan and how to individualize teaching for a particular patient or group. For example, discharge teaching has a different focus if the patient is discharged home alone, discharged home with a caregiver, or transferred to an extended-care facility. Teaching is especially important in the current healthcare environment because many errors and mistakes are made as patients transition from one level of health care to another. Some of these errors can be avoided with good patient teaching.

Example Using "Teaching Others" in Everyday Life

Teaching and learning occur at all stages of life. The formal school environment provides role models about how to teach. Informal environments such as within the family unit or clubs and organizations provide other times in life to experience teaching—both as a teacher and as a learner. Common examples of teaching others in everyday life include teaching a group of children in a church setting, teaching tasks to siblings, or training a new employee.

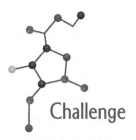

Challenge

Provide an example of how you use the critical thinking skill of "Teaching Others" in your everyday life.

_____

_____

_____

_____

_____

_____

_____

_____

_____

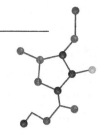

Nurses consider all factors, looking at the complete patient situation, to determine what to include in the teaching plan and how to individualize teaching for a particular patient or group.

Example Using "Teaching Others" in Nursing

Nurses are constantly teaching. They teach patients, other healthcare providers, and unlicensed assistive personnel. Some of the teaching is formal such as preoperative teaching for a patient scheduled for surgery or discharge teaching for the patient transferring to another healthcare environment or returning home. Nurses also teach other nurses about nursing procedures and interventions. Teaching is a major responsibility for nurses.

Reflecting Step

As mentioned earlier in this book, reflecting on your experience is required for learning and growing to occur. Merely having an experience isn't enough; you must think back and consider what occurred, what you learned from the experience, and how to use your experience to improve or continue using good thinking. Therefore, reflective thinking is tantamount to learning and growing as a nurse. There are two types of reflection: reflection-in-action and reflection-on-action as explained in Chapter 2 of this book. Although there are two types of reflection, as a student or new graduate you will likely spend most of your reflection time in reflection-on-action.

Reflection-on-action occurs upon completion of the action. This step is critical to improving thinking. During this step, you mentally review what just happened to determine what went right and what went wrong. What you learn from the experience is used to improve your thinking abilities and your nursing knowledge base. Reviewing your thinking and its effectiveness encourages deeper understanding of your ability to think, supports self-evaluation, and, with honest reflection, fosters your ability to use critical thinking and clinical judgment. This is the actual learning from experience step. Without this reflection, it is difficult to learn from experience.

As you engage in reflective practice throughout your nursing program and throughout your nursing career, you will begin to engage in reflection-in-action. This type of reflection occurs while engaging in the work of a nurse. You will eventually achieve the ability to effectively reflect-in-action as you grow as a nurse.

There are two thinking skills and strategies in the Reflecting Step presented in this book:

1. Evaluating data

2. Evaluating and correcting thinking

> Reviewing your thinking
> and its effectiveness
> encourages deeper
> understanding of your
> ability to think,
> supports self-evaluation,
> and, with honest reflection,
> fosters your ability
> to use critical thinking
> and clinical judgment.

EVALUATING DATA

Definition

Once actions have been performed, assessment data are again collected. These assessment data are used as the basis for determining if the interventions were effective. Accurate and complete data collection at this point provides a basis on which to determine what actions must be taken next. Questions that guide your thinking while evaluating data include:

- Have you collected all necessary data to determine the effectiveness of your interventions?

- Do you need to collect additional data?

- Do the data indicate the problem has been solved?

- Is the problem remaining constant so you will continue to implement the same strategies?

- Has a new problem arisen?

These and other questions are addressed at this time. The results of data evaluation provide the basis for determining what further actions are needed.

Example Using "Evaluating Data" in Everyday Life

This thinking skill is used continuously in everyday life, often unconsciously. For example, after making a new recipe for dinner you might evaluate how it tastes and determine what seemed to work the best or how to improve the recipe for a later time (a little more or a little less of a certain ingredient).

As another example, coaches of children's sport teams collect data about how each player performed, determine if additional information is needed, then decide how to help each child improve for the next game.

Challenge

Provide an example of how you use the critical thinking skill of "Evaluating Data" in your everyday life.

_____

_____

_____

_____

_____

_____

_____

_____

_____

_____

The results of
data evaluation
provide the basis for
determining what
further actions
are needed.

Example Using "Evaluating Data" in Nursing

Evaluating data is a major step in the nursing process. This thinking skill is critical to proper implementation of that step. Nurses collect data on an initial encounter with the patient. Interventions are planned and performed. At an appropriate time, the nurse returns to the patient to collect data to determine the effectiveness of the interventions. The evaluation data are used to determine if each intervention was effective. After evaluating the data, the nurse then makes further plans such as to continue the intervention, change the timing of the intervention, or even eliminate that intervention from the plan of care. This same process is used when evaluating actions related to handling a problem in the healthcare setting.

EVALUATING AND CORRECTING THINKING

Definition

After using critical thinking/clinical reasoning to resolve a problem, make a decision, or plan patient care, it is important to evaluate the thinking that occurred. Evaluating data, the previous thinking skill, helps the nurse determine if the actions were effective. This step is different because it evaluates the thinking used. This step requires reflecting on what just happened, how the situation was handled, and what lessons can be learned—that is, was the thinking faulty or was the thinking correct? Therefore, both evaluating data and evaluating thinking are critical processes to use to provide safe, effective nursing care and to grow as a nurse.

This type of self-evaluation about the thinking processes used promotes professional development, enhances self-esteem, fosters insight into one's own thinking, and promotes better clinical judgment/clinical reasoning in the future. Thinking about one's thinking is part of the total critical thinking process. Example questions that may be used to evaluate thinking include:

- What thinking skills were used? Were they effective?

- Were the outcomes what was expected? If not, were the outcomes acceptable or perhaps better than expected? If the outcomes were not acceptable, what might be done differently in the future?

- How did the thinking impact all the people affected, such as the patient, significant others, and other healthcare providers? Was the impact positive or negative?

It is helpful to discuss your thinking (debrief) with your teacher/preceptor. Ask if they would have handled the situation differently. Be ready to change if change is needed.

Example Using "Evaluating and Correcting Thinking" in Everyday Life

There are many times in everyday life when it is necessary to consider the thinking used to solve a problem. An example might be determining an approach to dealing with an issue with a child. Parents often face an undesirable behavior of a child. To deal with the behavior, the parents look at the situation and apply many thinking skills such as:

- Gathering accurate information

- Clustering related information

- Collaborating with each other or outside counsel

- Communicating with the child about the plan of action

Once implemented the parents gather data about how the child responded and if the thinking used led to improved behavior. Perhaps the evaluation data reveal additional thinking skills would have been helpful such as comparing and contrasting various approaches rather than considering just one.

Although many parents use these thinking skills to perfect parenting skills, articulation of this process if often missing. It is helpful in everyday life, just as it is in nursing, to be aware of thinking processes used and ways to improve.

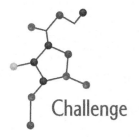

Challenge

Provide an example of how you use the critical thinking skill of "Evaluating and Correcting Thinking" in your everyday life.

_____

_____

_____

_____

_____

_____

_____

_____

_____

_____

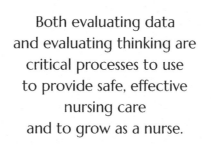

Both evaluating data
and evaluating thinking are
critical processes to use
to provide safe, effective
nursing care
and to grow as a nurse.

Example Using "Evaluating and Correcting Thinking" in Nursing

As nurses evaluate data as explained in the previous thinking skill "Evaluating Data", all expected and unexpected findings are analyzed. If a finding represents faulty thinking that led to a negative outcome the nurse must review the thinking that occurred and identify what went wrong. For example:

> *The nurse notices a patient's call light is on. The nurse is not directly caring for this patient but enters the patient's room to determine what the patient might need. The patient states he has an urgent need to use the bathroom and requires help to quickly walk to the bathroom. The nurse immediately helps the patient out of bed and begins walking the patient to the bathroom. With the second step the patient falls to the floor and yells, "Don't you know my right side is weak from a stroke I had three years ago!" The nurse immediately takes action to help the patient.*

Upon reflecting on this action, the nurse must determine what went wrong with the thinking used to plan the intervention of ambulating the patient. The nurse immediately identified not using the thinking skill of "Determining Important Information to Collect". Because the patient was alert and able to talk with the nurse, the nurse could have easily asked the patient if he had any problems or needed any special assistance ambulating. Once that important information was collected the nurse would have used the thinking skills of "Predicting Potential Complications" (falling) and "Managing Potential Complications". To manage the potential complication of falling the nurse might have:

1. Decided there wasn't enough time to ambulate the patient to the bathroom due to his weakness and offer him a bed pan.

2. Determined how to support the patient's weak side to safely ambulate him to the bathroom.

This is a very simple situation to analyze but demonstrates the importance of good thinking skills and the ability to apply them as a nurse.

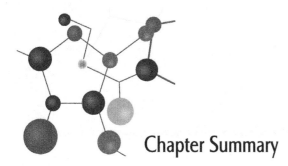

Chapter Summary

Chapter 4 introduced all the thinking skills used in this book for each of the four steps of the Clinical Judgment Model. Examples provided everyday use of each thinking skill as well as application to nursing.

The next step in your **development** of clinical judgment/clinical reasoning is using each of those thinking skills in actual nursing practice. The next chapter provides practice activities using each thinking skill as a nurse.

The activities provide guidance on how to use each thinking skill but also give you insight into the thinking processes you are using. This encourages the development of metacognition which means you are aware of your thinking processes and can explain them to others. This is an extremely important and useful skill to acquire.

CHAPTER 5

Beginning Level Thinking Activities

This chapter provides activities for you to use to apply and experience the use of thinking skills in nursing practice. You might consider these thinking activities as **clinical coaches** that help you navigate through patient situations in the complex healthcare environment, guiding you as you engage in higher and higher levels of thinking. In other words, the activities provide situated thinking, using knowledge to solve problems and applying clinical judgment to guide thinking. Coaching is further enhanced as you debrief your work using these activities with your clinical teacher/preceptor. The closer the time of debriefing with your teacher/preceptor to your completion of the activity, the more beneficial to your learning. Feedback provided in real time as soon as the clinical encounter occurs helps you improve your thinking (Jessee & Tanner, 2016). Feedback that is provided long after the clinical experience and completion of these activities is much less effective in facilitating learning (McNelis, et al., 2014).

These activities help you sort through all the "clinical noise" to determine what clinical knowledge and clinical data are relevant in an actual situation then determine how to use that knowledge to care for a specific patient. The notion of a "specific" patient is very important. There are many sources for "standardized" patient care in the form of pre-developed care plans for various patient situations. These care plans do not provide individualized or patient-centered care specific to a patient. Patient-centered care is a hallmark of current nursing practice. As a nurse, you may use research-based generalizations, but you are required to apply these generalizations to a particular patient's condition/situation, which can present unique circumstances not accounted for in the pre-developed care plans. It is only through quality clinical judgment/clinical reasoning that individual patient outcomes are improved; and, as previously stated, this is the overarching goal of nursing practice—improving patient outcomes.

Keep in mind that although each activity focuses on one thinking skill, to complete the activity you likely will use a number of other thinking skills. In most cases one thinking skill is not used in isolation. However, the purpose of these activities is to focus on one particular thinking skill to demonstrate its application to nursing practice.

> Patient-centered care is a hallmark of current nursing practice.

Noticing Step

As discussed in Chapter 2, the Noticing Step involves collecting data about the patient or other health-care situation. The nurse uses assessment techniques such as observation and auscultation to collect data. Additionally, an important skill to use during noticing is thoughtful questioning used to explore all aspects of the situation. During the Noticing Step the nurse notices that something is different than what was expected. Something doesn't seem right. For example, the nurse assesses the patient and discovers new information that was not included in the report received from the nurse on the previous shift or the nurse from a transferring unit or other healthcare facility. Or, perhaps the nurse understands the typical presenta-tion of a patient with a particular medical diagnosis, but the current patient demonstrates a variation from what is expected.

Because nurses also face issues and problems in the healthcare environment, this is also an aspect of nursing that requires attention. Nurses not only engage in nursing, but they also work to improve nursing. The safety of the healthcare environment is basic to safe patient care.

Following are basic tools to apply in the clinical setting to provide practice using the thinking skills used in the Noticing Step of the Clinical Judgment Model.

> Nurses not only engage in nursing, but they also work to improve nursing. The safety of the healthcare environment is basic to safe patient care.

IDENTIFYING SIGNS AND SYMPTOMS

This tool guides your use of the critical thinking skill of identifying signs and symptoms. There are many times you will use this thinking skill in many situations. The thinking in this tool is just one example.

Activity/Tool

The first step in identifying signs and symptoms is to gather information. To gather information, address each of the following:

1. What is the condition/situation/issue you are assessing to determine the presence of signs and symptoms you will later use to determine any variances (data out of the normal range or expectation). The condition/situation may be a medical diagnosis such as acute asthma or a specific issue such as fever. It may also be identifying the signs and symptoms about a concept such as perfusion or safety.

    _____

    _____

    _____

    _____

    _____

2. Answer the following questions about your knowledge base related to this condition/situation/issue:

    What do you know about this condition/situation/issue?

    _____

    _____

    _____

    _____

    _____

What do you need to review in a reference book prior to assessing the patient to identify signs and symptoms?

_____

_____

_____

_____

_____

What information will you collect and what sources will you use to gather the needed information?

Report from the nurse on the previous shift

_____

_____

_____

_____

_____

The patient's chart

~LAB RESULTS

_____

_____

_____

_____

_____

~PREVIOUS NURSE'S CHARTING (LAST 24 HOURS)

_____

_____

_____

_____

~OTHER INFORMATION FROM THE CHART

_____

_____

_____

_____

Patient assessment

_____

_____

_____

_____

Equipment in the room such as monitors, pumps, etc.

_____

_____

_____

_____

After you have gathered all the information you will identify signs and symptoms. Complete the following table.

Data Collected	Normal or expected findings for the condition/situation/ issue being assessed	Which patient data are outside of the normal range or expected findings that indicate an issue/ problem that needs to be addressed?

At this point in your thinking process you are concerned with:

1. Knowing what data to collect.

2. Ensuring you collect all pertinent data to identify any issues or problems.

3. Noticing signs and symptoms that are out of range or outside the normal expectations that you will later use to determine how you will respond.

As you become more experienced you will learn about tools that are available for identifying signs and symptoms about many patient care issues. For example, there are tools for assessing pain level and ones that assess a patient's risk to fall.

As suggested by the activities of this tool, you must be able to determine what information to collect, how to augment your knowledge base as needed, and sources of information that will yield the desired information.

Assessing Systematically and Comprehensively

Nurses use many tools to ensure data collection is systematic and comprehensive for the purpose of gathering all necessary data. One example of a systematic and comprehensive approach to data collection is an assessment of a patient's level of pain. The tool contains characteristics of pain that are important to consider when determining nursing interventions. This tool guides your thinking to ensure a systematic and comprehensive approach to data collection.

> In nursing, "assessing systematically and comprehensively" is defined as assessing patients using a systematic method such as a body systems or a head-to-toe approach so no areas are missed.

Activity/Tool

This tool is used to systematically and comprehensively collect both subjective and objective data. The patient's report about pain characteristics is subjective data. Objective data are also collected such as medications prescribed and the patient's history. This tool is expanded in Chapter 6 to include further objective data such as vital signs and other data. The tool in this chapter is an introduction.

_____ Assessing Pain

Location of pain:

_____

_____

Intensity:
(numeric rating 0 to 10)
0 = no pain
10 = worst pain possible

_____

Quality:
(What it feels like such as stabbing, burning, dull?)

_____

_____

Onset and duration:
(When did it start and how long does it last?)

_____

_____

Alleviating and relieving factors:
(What lessens the pain or relieves the pain?)

_____

_____

Effect of pain on function:
(Does the pain interfere with the patient's ability to perform normal activities?)

_____

_____

_____

_____

_____

_____

_____

Pain goal:
(What pain rating would the patient like to achieve?)

_____

_____

Other information, such as patient's culture, past pain experiences, and pertinent medical history related to pain:

_____

_____

_____

_____

_____

_____

MEDICATIONS
(focusing on pain medications)

Medication and dose
the patient is taking:

_____

_____

Frequency taking the
medication:

_____

Pain rating prior to receiving
the medication and the
patient's pain rating
30 minutes after receiving
the medication:

_____

_____

The patient's evaluation/
perception of the
effectiveness of the
medication:

_____

_____

_____

Any side effects or
untoward effects the
patient is experiencing:

_____

_____

_____

Other observations about
the patient and the
patient's pain:

_____

_____

_____

This systematic and comprehensive pain assessment yields important information necessary for planning the patient's care related to pain. This is one example of a tool focused on one area of nursing care. As you learn about nursing related to many other patient care issues, develop your own tools to guide your approach to a systematic and comprehensive assessment. The more you use your own developed tools, the more autonomous your assessment will become and the less reliant you will be on formalized tools such as these.

~That is the goal—making your thinking automatic!~

GATHERING ACCURATE INFORMATION

Any information gathered about patients or a problem in the healthcare setting must be accurate. Using inaccurate information can lead to poor patient outcomes. For example, using the wrong size blood pressure cuff can result in a wrong blood pressure reading. A patient's blood pressure medication may be given or held based on that inaccurate reading. It is critical that all data are accurate.

Nurses use many types of equipment to gather patient data. Ensuring the equipment is right for the job and that the equipment is working correctly gives the nurse confidence in the accuracy of the data collected.

Activity/Tool

Conduct an inventory of the equipment on the clinical unit used to measure and collect patient data. Add that equipment to the left column of the table. In the right column explain how you will ensure the equipment is what is needed for the patient and/or that the equipment is functioning properly. Some equipment is already listed.

Equipment used to collect patient data	How you will ensure you are using the right piece of equipment and that the equipment is functioning properly
Electronic Thermometer	
Blood Pressure Cuff	
Glucose Meter	

Add more equipment present on the clinical unit

PREDICTING POTENTIAL COMPLICATIONS

This tool helps you determine potential complications that may occur. It is important you think about these because it is the nurse's responsibility to keep the patient safe. This is part of using clinical forethought as discussed earlier in this book. Clinical forethought was previously discussed in the context of anticipating what might go wrong during a nursing intervention. Predicting potential complications related to the individual patient situation is another application of clinical forethought. These complications not only relate to the patient's medical diagnosis, but also to individual factors about that patient. Following are some individual factors that may put the patient at risk for a potential complication in addition to the medical diagnosis or surgical procedure.

- Is there anything about this patient that leads you to believe there is a possibility the patient might fall?

- Is the patient physically weak and need assistance ambulating?

- Is the patient 65 years of age or older and at risk to fall?

- Is the patient cognitively impaired and not able to follow instructions?

- Does the patient have a sensory loss such as poor hearing or vision?

- Is the patient taking medications that cause dizziness or make the patient drowsy?

Activity/Tool

Based on your current level of nursing knowledge, answer the following questions related to your patient.

1. What are you on alert for today with this patient and why?

    _____

    _____

2. What are the important assessments to make and why?

    _____

    _____

3. What complications may occur and why?

    _____

    _____

4. Based on the above, what could go wrong?

    _____

    _____

After completing the above, go to the thinking skill of Managing Potential Complications under the Interpreting Step to plan what you will do for this patient.

Interpreting Step

As discussed in Chapter 2 the thinking skills used in the Noticing Step yield information about the patient or situation. The Interpreting Step requires you to analyze the data to make sense of all the data collected. In the Interpreting Step, you sort through the information collected, analyze the information, and use it to develop a plan. The thinking skills and strategies used in this step help answer questions such as:

- What do the data mean?

- How should the data be interpreted for this patient?

- What are the most important data?

- What actions should be planned?

- How should the actions be prioritized?

Therefore, in the Interpreting Step your goal is to:

- Process the information you "noticed"—data collected related to the patient and the healthcare environment.

- Analyze that data to come to a clear, accurate understanding of the situation.

- Based on your understanding of the situation, determine actions you will take.

The end product of the Interpreting Step is your plan; how you will care for the patient or handle an issue in the healthcare setting. Following are basic tools to apply in the clinical setting to provide practice using the thinking skills used in the Interpreting Step of the Clinical Judgment Model.

CLUSTERING RELATED INFORMATION

One of the most important responsibilities of a nurse is to keep the patient safe. Safety is a very important concept that has many dimensions. There are observable factors to assess such as environmental conditions related to cluttered walkways or water on the floor. Other factors may not be so obvious. Generally, ensuring safety requires collecting a variety of types of information that are clustered together to determine risks to the patient's safety. This tool guides your thinking about patient safety.

Activity/Tool

_____ Patient Safety

Age:

Language:

Language barriers:

Physical strength:

Physical limitations:

Level of consciousness:

Cognitive ability:
(Can the patient understand instructions, read signs, understand what the signs mean, etc.?)

_____

_____

_____

_____

Effects the disease process may have on safety and explain:

_____

_____

_____

_____

Effects of medications on safety specific for this patient and explain:

_____

_____

_____

_____

_____

Environment:

_____

_____

_____

Tubes:

_____

_____

_____

Equipment:

_____

_____

_____

Assistance available to help
the patient:

_____

_____

Identification band on?

_____

Allergy band on?

_____

Current information
on the patient board:

_____

Call light available:

_____

Add any further information
or precautions you identified
that are specific for this
patient:

_____

_____

_____

The nurse considers all these factors and uses this information to plan interventions to keep the patient safe. Based on the above information you collected, list the information that indicates a potential safety issue for this patient and plan interventions to ensure safety.

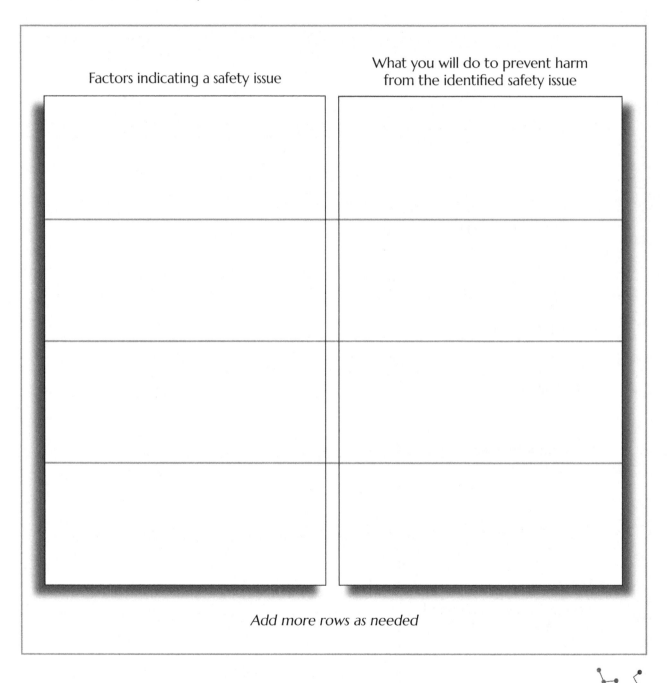

Factors indicating a safety issue	What you will do to prevent harm from the identified safety issue

Add more rows as needed

RECOGNIZING INCONSISTENCIES

As nurses work with patients they are constantly comparing patient information to what is expected based on:

- The nurse's level of knowledge

- Agency guidelines

- Evidence-based practice standards

Often there appears to be inconsistencies between the patient's presentation and that which is expected from standard protocol. Two reasons for variances are:

1. There is something unique about this patient that requires a change to the normal protocol or approach.

2. Something may have been missed or an error was made.

Both these reasons must be considered. The nurse must understand any variances based on sound rationale considering each patient as unique. However, if something was missed or an error made, the nurse must take action to correct the situation.

> In reviewing the data, nurses use the thinking skill of recognizing inconsistencies among all the subjective and the objective data that may indicate additional problems that are not readily apparent.

Activity/Tool

This activity requires you to compare and contrast information to identify any inconsistencies. Complete the following table.

1	2	3	4
What is medically prescribed and/or nursing inventions for this patient	Textbook expectations regarding medical orders and nursing interventions	Agency guidelines or other evidence-based sources (cite source)	Differences or variances between what is ordered or planned and what is indicated in the text-book, agency guidelines, or other sources

Add more rows as needed

Discuss each item listed in Column 4. Explain why there is a variance and if there are any actions the nurse must take related to that variance.

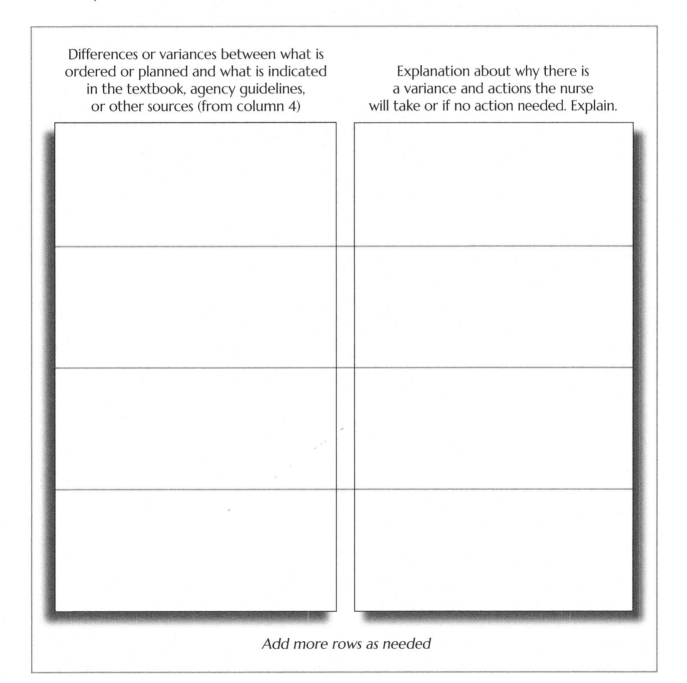

Differences or variances between what is ordered or planned and what is indicated in the textbook, agency guidelines, or other sources (from column 4)	Explanation about why there is a variance and actions the nurse will take or if no action needed. Explain.

Add more rows as needed

DETERMINING IMPORTANT INFORMATION TO COLLECT AND DISTINGUISHING RELEVANT FROM IRRELEVANT INFORMATION

The thinking skills of Determining Important Information to Collect and Distinguishing Relevant from Irrelevant Information appear to be similar and they are. Remember, when learning about these thinking skills and engaging in practice using them, it is necessary to separate them out or "unpack" them. However, when engaging in nursing practice you will use many thinking skills, selecting out the ones you will use in any given situation.

When you approach a patient situation you must sort through the myriad of information to consider when planning care for that patient. You must determine what information is important to collect and what information is not important for that particular patient situation. Once you have collected all the important information that is necessary for you to provide safe, quality nursing care, you then use the critical thinking skill of "Distinguishing Relevant From Irrelevant Information". That is, which data that you collected are relevant that you must act on when you consider that data within the bigger picture of the patient. The next two activities provide practice with these thinking skills.

DETERMINING IMPORTANT INFORMATION TO COLLECT

When caring for a patient with whom you are unfamiliar, you will collect much information about the patient. That information provides a total patient picture (Determining Important Information to Collect). From there you consider the specific information about that patient and what is happening with the patient at the current time to determine what information indicates a need for action (Distinguishing Relevant from Irrelevant Information).

You must determine
what information
is important
to collect for
each patient.

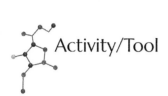 Activity/Tool

_____ Patient Information

Collect the following information about your patient:

Age:

_____

Reason for admission:

_____

Date of admission:

_____

Diagnostic procedures:

_____

_____

Surgical procedure:

_____

_____

Diet:

_____

_____

Activity:

_____

_____

Vital signs:

_____

Trending of vital signs:
*(How have the vital signs
changed from the previous
reading; from the previous
24 hours?)*

_____

_____

_____

MEDICATIONS

Drug:

_____

_____

Reason drug was prescribed:

_____

_____

Therapeutic effects expected:

_____

_____

Adverse effects to monitor:

_____

_____

What results did the
patient experience?

_____

_____

_____

Complete for each medication prescribed.

PATIENT HISTORY

Review patient's history:
(From the history, determine the most important data impacting this hospitalization.)

_____

_____

_____

_____

DIAGNOSTIC TESTS

Name of test:

_____

Why was this test ordered?

_____

_____

_____

Test results:

_____

_____

_____

Trending of the results:
(If the test was performed more than once, how have the results changed from the previous readings?)

_____

_____

_____

Complete for each test ordered.

Was all the information you noted important to collect for this patient?

Why?

Why not?

Is there other information not included in the list that you should review? List that information and explain why it would be important to review that information as well.

Answer the following questions:

_____

_____

_____

_____

_____

_____

_____

_____

_____

_____

_____

_____

_____

_____

_____

_____

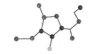

Distinguishing Relevant from Irrelevant Information

Look at the data you collected from the activity for the thinking skill "Determining Important Information to Collect." Review the data to determine which data are relevant to the care of the patient on this day. All the information may be important, but your task now is to distinguish which data are relevant and how that data will influence the care you provide for this patient today.

Activity/Tool

For the information you recorded for the thinking skill "Determining Important Information to Collect" indicate the relevant data. Insert that information in the table below in the first column. In the second column discuss why that data are relevant for the current, immediate care of this patient.

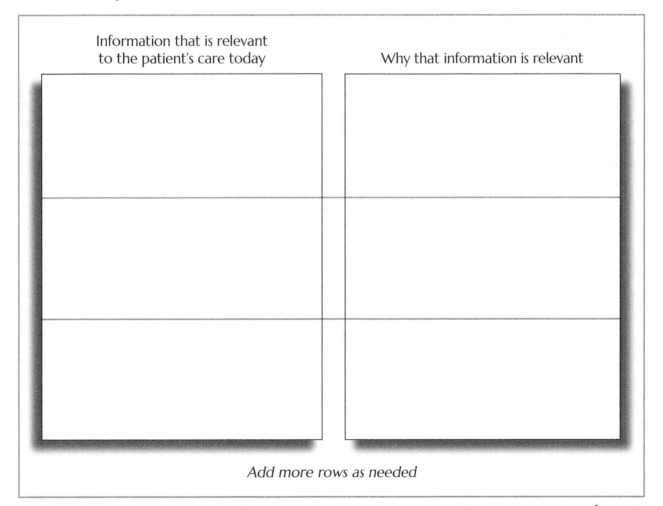

Information that is relevant to the patient's care today	Why that information is relevant

Add more rows as needed

Remember, although all the information was important to review, only some of the data are relevant for planning care for this day. Consider the following approach:

- Are there findings present now that were not previously apparent?

- Are there data that indicate a problem is developing or is present?

- Examine data that have changed from previous readings. Are those changes indicative of the patient improving? Are those data indicative of the patient's condition worsening?

- Are the medications working? What tells you yes or what tells you no?

JUDGING HOW MUCH AMBIGUITY IS ACCEPTABLE

The purpose of this activity is to experience how nurses think through a specific patient situation; that is, considering a rule such as "within normal limits" to a specific patient situation to determine how much wiggle room is acceptable. This activity applies the specific thinking skill of judging how much ambiguity is acceptable when considering a patient's vital signs.

Nurses must collect data, analyze the data, and determine the importance of the information, all within the context of the patient, then they can determine how to apply the rules they learned about "within normal limits" for vital signs. The "within the context of the patient" is where the thinking skill of judging how much ambiguity (wiggle room) is acceptable applies. However, it is difficult to witness how a nurse uses this thinking skill because it is done so quickly and automatically.

> Nurses determine how
> to apply rules they
> learned about information
> within the context of
> the patient.

Activity/Tool

The purpose of this tool is to guide you through the process with a step-by-step approach applied to one area of patient care.

_____Patient's Vital Signs

What are the patient's current vital signs?

Blood pressure:

_____

Pulse:

_____

Respirations:

_____

Temperature:

_____

What are the vital signs for the past 24 hours?

_____

_____

_____

What are the highs and lows for the past 24 hours?

_____

_____

_____

Is the patient experiencing pain? If so, what is the patient's pain level based on a scale of 0 to 10?

_____

_____

_____

What is the patient's activity level?

_____

_____

_____

What medications is the patient taking that affect the vital signs? Describe the effect of each medication on each of the vital signs.

_____

_____

_____

_____

What medical/nursing interventions is the patient experiencing that may affect the patient's vital signs?

_____

_____

_____

What other factors are influencing this patient's vital sign readings?

_____

_____

_____

How low can each of the
readings go before you
would intervene?
Give your rationale.

_____

_____

_____

_____

How high can each of the
readings go before you
would intervene?
Give your rationale.

_____

_____

_____

_____

Are the current vital signs
acceptable for this patient?
Explain.

_____

_____

_____

_____

The purpose of this assignment is not to teach a list of steps to memorize when considering a patient's vital signs. The purpose of the assignment is to use a specific critical thinking skill to analyze data to arrive at a decision based on the specific patient situation, or the context of the patient. This provides practice understanding that decisions are made not based on individual pieces of information, but within the specific patient context. The amount of ambiguity that can be tolerated for one patient may be quite different for another.

COMPARING AND CONTRASTING

Comparing and contrasting patients with similar situations helps the nurse discover the nuances, or small differences, among the patients. Although these differences may be small, the differences may greatly influence the decisions you make.

Activity/Tool

_____ Patient Information

For each of 3 patients who have been diagnosed with an infection, collect the following information:

Age:

_____

Number of days in hospital:

_____

Medical diagnosis:

_____

_____

_____

Pre-existing conditions:

_____

_____

_____

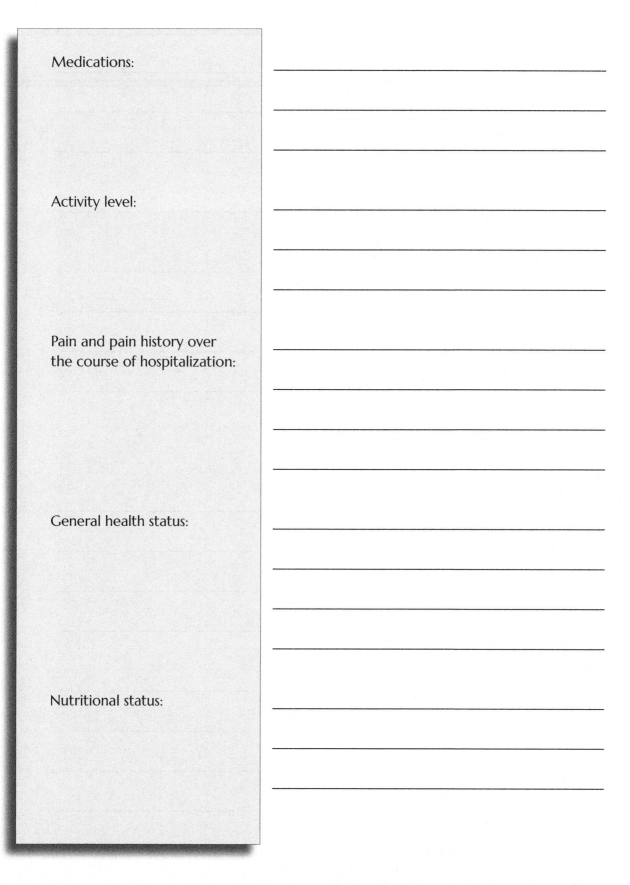

Medications:

Activity level:

Pain and pain history over
the course of hospitalization:

General health status:

Nutritional status:

Hydration status:

_____

_____

_____

Lifestyle including:

_____

~nutritional intake

_____

~tobacco use

_____

~alcohol intake

_____

~substance abuse

_____

INFECTION PRESENT

Type and location
of infection:

_____

_____

_____

_____

Assessment related to
existing infection:

_____

_____

_____

_____

Course of treatment:

_____

_____

_____

Compare and Contrast Data for the Three Patients

How are the infections
the same? Different?

_____

_____

_____

How are the treatments
the same? Different?

_____

_____

_____

How is each responding
to treatment?

_____

_____

_____

Which factors are most
influential for each of the
patient's recovery from
the infection?

_____

_____

_____

MANAGING POTENTIAL COMPLICATIONS

Review the assignment you completed for the thinking skill **"Predicting Potential Complications"**. Use that information to complete the following thinking tool.

Activity/Tool

For each of the potential complications you identified, plan interventions to prevent those complications from occurring.

Potential Complication	Interventions to PREVENT the potential complication from occurring

Add more rows as needed

Explain what you will do if each of the complications does occur.

Potential Complication	What you will do should the complication occur

Add more rows as needed

IDENTIFYING ASSUMPTION

Activity/Tool

Review the information you received from the nurse about your patient. Prior to visiting your patient complete the following table.

Information about this patient	What I know about this information	Assumptions about the patient I can make based on this information
Age		
Culture		
Religion		
Developmental Level		
Socioeconomic Status		
Type of Health Insurance		
Other Information Unique to this Patient		

Now visit the patient. Ensuring sensitivity, during your conversation gather data from the patient about each of the factors listed in the table.

Complete the following table.

Information I collected from this patient about each factor	Identify differences from your assumptions prior to visiting the patient to what you learned while visiting the patient
Age	
Culture	
Religion	
Developmental Level	
Socioeconomic Status	
Type of Health Insurance	
Other Information Unique to this Patient	

Discuss the results of your analysis of assumptions. Talk about how those assumptions might influence the care you provide.

_____

_____

_____

_____

_____

_____

_____

_____

Discuss what you learned from this activity.

_____

_____

_____

_____

_____

_____

_____

_____

SETTING PRIORITIES

There are a number of ways nurses set priorities. This tool uses what is known as the ABCD Prioritization Model:

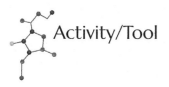 Activity/Tool

- A (absolutely now)

- B (better get to in the first hour)

- C (can wait for a few hours)

- D (can delegate)

_____ Prioritization Form

Review your plan of care for the day. After assessing your patient, use this prioritization model to answer these questions:

What nursing interventions are needed for your patient today?

_____

_____

_____

_____

What interventions do you consider in the A group (absolutely now)? Explain.

_____

_____

_____

_____

What complications may occur if you do not carry out immediately the interventions in the A group?

_____

_____

_____

_____

What interventions do you consider in the B group (better get to in the first hour)? Explain.

_____

_____

_____

_____

What complications may occur if you do not carry out these interventions within the first hour?

_____

_____

_____

What interventions do you consider in the C group (can wait for a few hours)? Explain.

_____

_____

_____

What interventions do you consider in the D group (can delegate)? Explain.

_____

_____

_____

COLLABORATING WITH OTHER HEALTHCARE TEAM MEMBERS

As you work through your day think about aspects of your patient care that require you to collaborate with other healthcare team members. Complete the following table with that information.

Activity/Tool

Which member of the healthcare team will you communicate with?	What information will you share?	What information do you expect to receive from this team member?	Actual collaboration you carried out.	Ways to improve communication while collaborating with other healthcare team members.

Add more rows as needed

Responding Step

As discussed in Chapter 2, the determinations made in the Interpreting Step are important for deciding how, and to what degree, you will respond. After planning actions to take, but prior to implementing the actions in the Responding Step, always think ahead and consider what you expect to happen when you implement your plan. Think about what should go right and what could go wrong. Always have a plan for what to do should something go wrong. This is extremely important. Clinical forethought—thinking ahead about what might happen in a clinical situation—is very important during the Responding Step.

Following are basic tools to apply in the clinical setting to provide practice using the thinking skills used in the Responding Step of the Clinical Judgment Model.

DELEGATING

As you learn about nursing you will discover there is a process that is used to guide the nurse when delegating. A critical component of that process is knowing what task can be delegated. Registered Nurses delegate nursing tasks to an LPN/LVN or to an unlicensed assistive person such as a Certified Nursing Assistant (CNA). The LPN/LVN can also delegate tasks in many states; however, in some states the LPN/LVN makes assignments rather than delegates.

Two important documents that provide the basis about who can delegate and to whom to delegate are the nurse practice act for your state and the agency's job descriptions for RN, LPN/LVN, and unlicensed assistive personnel.

> Clinical forethought—
> thinking ahead about what
> might happen in a
> clinical situation—
> is very important
> during the
> Responding Step.

Activity/Tool

To complete this activity you will need a copy of your state's nurse practice act that discusses scope of practice of the RN and the LPN/LVN and the agency's job descriptions. Use the information in these documents for your "because" explanations in the second and third columns.

Nursing Intervention	I can delegate this intervention to an LPN/LVN because...	I can delegate this intervention to a CNA because...

Add more rows as needed

COMMUNICATING

The purpose of this activity is to provide practice using therapeutic communication techniques when communicating with patients and their families. You will need a list of the therapeutic communication techniques you learned in a fundamentals of nursing course or a mental health nursing course. Take that list to the clinical setting.

Activity/Tool

After interacting with a patient, leave the room and immediately complete the following table.

Therapeutic communication techniques used with patient	Example of using the therapeutic communication technique	How the communication was effective	How the communication was ineffective	Ways you can improve

Add more rows as needed

Were you able to identify the therapeutic communication techniques you used?

_____

_____

_____

_____

_____

_____

How will you use this experience to improve communication with the patient and family?

_____

_____

_____

_____

_____

_____

TEACHING OTHERS

A major responsibility of the nurse is to teach. Those you teach can include patients, their families, and other healthcare providers. This activity involves teaching patients. Visit your patient and/or the patient's family. Collect information about the patient based on each of the areas listed in the table below.

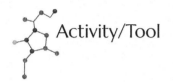 Activity/Tool

Areas to Assess	Assessment Information for this Patient
Educational Level	
Literacy Level	
Social Support	
Financial Resources	
Educational Resources	
Developmental Stage	
Hierarchy of Needs *(What might need to be addressed prior to starting the teaching)*	
Generational Differences	
Barriers to Learning	

After completing your assessment, identify what information is most important to consider when planning teaching for your patient by answering the following questions.

1. Which are the most important aspects to consider when planning teaching for this patient/family?

    _____

    _____

    _____

    _____

2. Using the information from the assessment table, how will you individualize your teaching? If this patient is a child, who will you teach in addition to the child such as a parent or guardian?

    _____

    _____

    _____

    _____

3. How will you know if your teaching was effective?

    _____

    _____

    _____

    _____

Reflecting Step

As discussed in Chapter 2, reflecting on your experience is required for learning and growing to occur. Merely having an experience isn't enough; you must think back and consider what occurred, what you can learn from it, and how to use your experience to improve, or continue using good thinking. Therefore, reflective thinking is tantamount to learning and growing as a nurse. Reviewing your thinking and its effectiveness encourages deeper understanding of your ability to think, supports self-evaluation, and, with honest reflection, fosters your ability to use critical thinking and clinical judgment/clinical reasoning.

Following are basic tools to apply in the clinical setting to provide practice applying the thinking skills used in the Reflecting Step of the Clinical Judgment Model.

EVALUATING DATA

Once the actions have been performed, assessment data are again collected. These assessment data are used as the basis for determining if the interventions were effective. Accurate and complete data collection at this point provides a basis on which to determine what actions must be taken next. This thinking skill looks at the answers to the following questions:

1. Have you collected all necessary data to determine the effectiveness of your interventions?

2. Do you need to collect additional data?

3. Do the data indicate the problem has been resolved?

4. Is the problem remaining constant so you will continue to implement the same strategies?

5. Has a new problem arisen?

These and other questions are addressed at this time. The results of the evaluation of data provide the basis for determining what further actions are needed.

> Reviewing your thinking and its effectiveness encourages deeper understanding of your ability to think, supports self-evaluation, and, with honest reflection, fosters your ability to use critical thinking and clinical judgment/clinical reasoning.

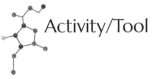 Activity/Tool

Assess your patient then complete the following tool.

Patient issue identified during your assessment	What interventions did you carry out for this patient r/t this issue or concern?	What evaluation data did you collect?	Are there new issues you need to address?	How will you revise the plan of care to incorporate un-resolved issues as well as additional issues identified as areas of concern?

Add more rows as needed

EVALUATING AND CORRECTING THINKING

As discussed earlier, after using clinical judgment/clinical reasoning to resolve a problem, make a decision, or plan patient care, it is important to evaluate the thinking that occurred. Evaluating data, the previous thinking skill, helps the nurse determine if the actions were effective. This step is different because it evaluates the **thinking** you used. This step requires reflecting on what just happened, how the situation was handled, and what lessons can be learned to improve your thinking.

Activity/Tool

After receiving feedback from your teacher/preceptor, complete the following tool.

Feedback from your teacher/preceptor about your thinking	Your impression of your thinking	How is your impression the same/different from that of your teacher/preceptor?	How will you use the feedback?
Add more rows as needed			

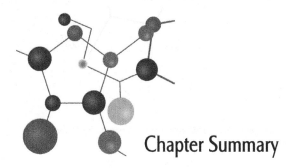

Chapter Summary

These tools provide basic, simple application of each of the thinking skills in each of the four steps of the Clinical Judgment Model. Continue using the thinking in these tools as you continue to care for patients and work within various healthcare settings.

The next chapter of this book builds on these thinking skills. The activities in Chapter 6 are more complex and require the use of several thinking skills. You will work through these activities and at the conclusion of each activity identify the thinking skills and strategies you used.

CHAPTER 6

Advanced Level Thinking Activities

This chapter provides advanced thinking activities for you to use. You may use these activities as you see fit. However, if you are new to nursing practice or if you have not learned clinical judgment/clinical reasoning in the manner in which it is taught in this book, you may want to first complete all the activities in Chapter 5.

These activities are different from the ones in Chapter 5 in a couple of important ways. First, these activities are not grouped according to a step in the Clinical Judgment Model. Second, the activities do not focus on a specific thinking skill. These activities require an in-depth look at a situation. The activities provide guidance in thinking using a number of thinking skills. Also, they are different than the activities in Chapter 5 because these activities require you to determine what thinking skills you used to complete the activity. Finally, you will explain the thinking skills you used. This analysis of your own thinking is called using metacognition. Metacognition refers to your ability to explain your thinking. Engaging in metacognition means you understand, analyze, and control your own cognitive processes. As your abilities in nursing practice grow so will your ability to engage in metacognition. The nurse who is able to engage in these higher levels of thinking is more able to provide safe, quality patient care and improve patient outcomes. Higher level thinking is also important when engaging in quality improvement to not only provide nursing care but to improve nursing care and to improve the safety and quality of the healthcare setting.

Pain Assessment

You used the below assessment as a beginning level tool for assessing systematically and comprehensively. This tool is presented again but this time is expanded with additional data to collect. In this advanced thinking assignment you use this expanded tool collecting data from three different patients. You examine the results of your assessment of three patients and identify differences or nuances. Although some differences or nuances may be subtle, they may influence the actions the nurse will take when planning individualized, patient-centered care.

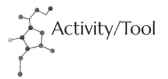
Activity/Tool

_____Assessing Pain

Note the following qualities of pain based on the data you collected and/or what is documented in the medical record for each of three patients:

Location of pain:

_____

_____

Intensity:
(numeric rating O to IO)
O = no pain
IO = worst pain possible

_____

Quality:
(What it feels like such as stabbing, burning, dull?)

_____

_____

Onset and duration:
(When did it start and how long does it last?)

_____

_____

Alleviating and relieving factors:
(What lessens the pain or relieves the pain?)

_____

_____

Effect of pain on function:
*(Does the pain interfere
with the patient's ability to
perform normal activities?)*

_____

_____

_____

_____

_____

_____

_____

_____

Pain goal:
*(What pain rating would
the patient like to achieve?)*

_____

Other information, such as
patient's culture, past pain
experiences, and pertinent
medical history related
to pain:

_____

_____

_____

_____

_____

_____

_____

MEDICATIONS
(focusing on pain medications)

Medication and dose
the patient is taking:

_____

_____

Frequency taking the
medication:

_____

Pain rating prior to receiving
the medication and the
patient's pain rating
30 minutes after receiving
the medication:

_____

_____

The patient's evaluation/
perception of the
effectiveness of the
medication:

_____

_____

_____

Any side effects or
untoward effects the
patient is experiencing:

_____

_____

_____

Other observations about
the patient and the
patient's pain:

_____

_____

_____

_____

PHYSIOLOGIC RESPONSES

Vital signs: _____

_____

Skin color: _____

Perspiration: _____

Pupil size: _____

Nausea: _____

Muscle tension: _____

Anxiety: _____

BEHAVIORAL RESPONSES

Posture, gross motor
activities: _____

Facial features: _____

Verbal expressions: _____

AFFECTIVE RESPONSES

Anxiety: _____

Depression: _____

Pattern of interacting
with others when the
pain is present: _____

Degree to which pain
interferes with ADLs/life: _____

_____

Perception of pain and
meaning to the patient: _____

Adaptive mechanisms used
to cope with the pain: _____

MEDICATIONS
(focusing on pain medications)

Medication and dose
the patient is taking: _____

_____

Frequency taking the
medication: _____

Pain rating prior to receiving the medication and the patient's pain rating 30 minutes after receiving the medication:

_____

_____

The patient's evaluation/ perception of the effectiveness of the medication:

_____

_____

_____

_____

Any side effects or untoward effects the patient is experiencing:

_____

_____

_____

_____

Other observations about the patient and the patient's pain:

_____

_____

_____

_____

_____

Analyze the data for the three patients answering the following questions:

How is each patient responding to the treatment for pain?

_____

_____

_____

_____

What factors are most influential in the patient's control of pain?

_____

_____

_____

Compare the medications for each patient. How are they the same? How are they different?

_____

_____

_____

_____

Why do different patients receive different pain medications?

_____

_____

_____

_____

What are some conclusions you can make about the differences among these three patients and how those differences influence the care the nurse will provide?

_____

_____

_____

_____

_____

_____

_____

_____

_____

_____

_____

_____

What thinking skills did you use? Use the following table to explain how you used each thinking skill.

Critical Thinking Skill/Strategy	Discuss which thinking skills were used and how each was used
NOTICING Identifying Signs and Symptoms Assessing Systematically and Comprehensively Gathering Accurate Data Predicting Potential Complications	
INTERPRETING Clustering Related Information Recognizing Inconsistencies Determining Important Information to Collect Distinguishing Relevant from Irrelevant Information Judging How Much Ambiguity is Acceptable Comparing and Contrasting Managing Potential Complications Identifying Assumptions Setting Priorities Collaborating with Other Healthcare Team Members	
RESPONDING Delegating Communicating Teaching Others	
REFLECTING Evaluating Data Evaluating and Correcting Thinking	

Predicting and Managing Potential Complications

These two thinking skills are combined in this advanced level activity. The purpose is to demonstrate the important connection between the two.

Activity/Tool

Assess three patients. Answer the following questions for each patient.

1. What are you on alert for today with this patient? (Predicting)

_____

_____

_____

_____

_____

_____

Explain why this is important.

_____

_____

_____

_____

_____

_____

2. What are the important assessments to make?   (Predicting)
    Explain why these assessments are important.

    _____

    _____

    _____

    _____

    _____

3. What complications may occur? What could go wrong? (Predicting)
    Relate the assessment data to the potential complication that may occur.

    _____

    _____

    _____

    _____

    _____

4. What interventions will prevent complications?   (Managing)
    Discuss how the interventions prevent complications.

    _____

    _____

    _____

    _____

    _____

5. What will you do if the complication does occur? (Managing)
    Explain how your planned interventions immediately treat, stop, or reverse
    the complication.

    _____

    _____

    _____

    _____

Discuss

1. What puts each patient at risk for each complication identified?

    _____

    _____

    _____

    _____

2. Why are there differences among the three patients?

    _____

    _____

    _____

    _____

In addition to the thinking skills of predicting and managing potential complications,
what thinking skills did you use? Use the following table to explain how you used
each thinking skill.

Critical Thinking Skill/Strategy	Discuss which thinking skills were used and how each was used
NOTICING Identifying Signs and Symptoms Assessing Systematically and Comprehensively Gathering Accurate Data Predicting Potential Complications	
INTERPRETING Clustering Related Information Recognizing Inconsistencies Determining Important Information to Collect Distinguishing Relevant from Irrelevant Information Judging How Much Ambiguity is Acceptable Comparing and Contrasting Managing Potential Complications Identifying Assumptions Setting Priorities Collaborating with Other Healthcare Team Members	
RESPONDING Delegating Communicating Teaching Others	
REFLECTING Evaluating Data Evaluating and Correcting Thinking	

National Patient Safety Goals

The National Patient Safety Goals (NPSGs) are a standard for ensuring basic safety for patients in different healthcare environments. Access the NPSGs for the healthcare environment in which you are working. These are available at: www.jointcommission.org/standards_information/npsgs.aspx

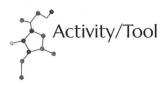

Activity/Tool

Using the NPSGs as a guide, answer the following questions.

1. What precautions should you take relative to each safety goal for your patient?

    _____

    _____

    _____

    _____

    _____

2. For your patient, is there a safety goal that is most relevant?

    _____

    _____

    _____

    _____

    _____

3. What factors about the environment indicate these safety goals are being met?

_____

_____

_____

_____

_____

4. What factors about the environment indicate a need for change so the safety goals can be met?

_____

_____

_____

_____

_____

5. How will you incorporate knowledge of the NPSGs into your practice as a nurse?

_____

_____

_____

_____

_____

What thinking skills did you use? Use the following table to explain how you used each thinking skill.

Critical Thinking Skill/Strategy	Discuss which thinking skills were used and how each was used
NOTICING Identifying Signs and Symptoms Assessing Systematically and Comprehensively Gathering Accurate Data Predicting Potential Complications	
INTERPRETING Clustering Related Information Recognizing Inconsistencies Determining Important Information to Collect Distinguishing Relevant from Irrelevant Information Judging How Much Ambiguity is Acceptable Comparing and Contrasting Managing Potential Complications Identifying Assumptions Setting Priorities Collaborating with Other Healthcare Team Members	
RESPONDING Delegating Communicating Teaching Others	
REFLECTING Evaluating Data Evaluating and Correcting Thinking	

Applying Thinking to Performing Nursing Skills

A list of steps is typically used when teaching/learning a specific nursing psychomotor skill. Novice nurses use that checklist to ensure all steps are performed. As the nurse's ability to look at each patient as an individual grows, it becomes apparent the specific order and approach to each step for performing a nursing skill may need to be modified. This activity requires you to look for relevant information about a patient situation that is used to influence how a particular nursing skill is performed.

Activity/Tool

This activity requires you to reference a nursing skills checklist for a skill of your choice. Review the checklist. Visit a patient and perform a head-to-assessment. Answer the following questions.

1. What information did you gather during the assessment that is important to consider when preparing to perform the skill? Explain.

    _____

    _____

    _____

    _____

2. Which data are relevant to the performance of the skill; that is, which data require you to modify the order of the steps of the skill as they are written? Explain.

    _____

    _____

    _____

    _____

3. Which data require you to modify the manner in which any of the steps of the skill are performed? Explain.

    _____

    _____

    _____

    _____

    _____

    _____

4. What precautions will you take to ensure the skill is performed with the modified approach without compromising patient safety? Explain.

    _____

    _____

    _____

    _____

    _____

    _____

What thinking skills did you use? Use the following table to explain how you used each thinking skill.

Critical Thinking Skill/Strategy	Discuss which thinking skills were used and how each was used
NOTICING Identifying Signs and Symptoms Assessing Systematically and Comprehensively Gathering Accurate Data Predicting Potential Complications	
INTERPRETING Clustering Related Information Recognizing Inconsistencies Determining Important Information to Collect Distinguishing Relevant from Irrelevant Information Judging How Much Ambiguity is Acceptable Comparing and Contrasting Managing Potential Complications Identifying Assumptions Setting Priorities Collaborating with Other Healthcare Team Members	
RESPONDING Delegating Communicating Teaching Others	
REFLECTING Evaluating Data Evaluating and Correcting Thinking	

Relevant Data on Which to Act

Review your patient's history and perform a patient assessment. Select the activity below which aligns with your patient.

Activity/Tool

Patient Undergoing Surgery

Read the patient's history and physical, including previous surgeries, medical history, and medications taken prior to admission. Discuss which information from the review of the patient's medical record and your assessment will have an impact on the patient's recovery from surgery. Explain the relationship between the patient information and recovery. For each piece of information determine which data are relevant to the care you will provide this day.

_____

_____

_____

_____

Patient Being Treated Medically

If the patient is being treated medically, discuss which information from the review of the patient's medical record and your assessment will have an impact on the patient's recovery from the current illness. Explain the relationship between the patient information and recovery. For each piece of information determine which data are relevant to the care you will provide this day.

_____

_____

_____

_____

What thinking skills did you use? Use the following table to explain how you used each thinking skill.

Critical Thinking Skill/Strategy	Discuss which thinking skills were used and how each was used
NOTICING Identifying Signs and Symptoms Assessing Systematically and Comprehensively Gathering Accurate Data Predicting Potential Complications	
INTERPRETING Clustering Related Information Recognizing Inconsistencies Determining Important Information to Collect Distinguishing Relevant from Irrelevant Information Judging How Much Ambiguity is Acceptable Comparing and Contrasting Managing Potential Complications Identifying Assumptions Setting Priorities Collaborating with Other Healthcare Team Members	
RESPONDING Delegating Communicating Teaching Others	
REFLECTING Evaluating Data Evaluating and Correcting Thinking	

What To Do with Data

Activity/Tool

Assess your patient. After your assessment answer the following questions.

What patient data did you collect?

_____

_____

_____

_____

What data are out of range?

_____

_____

_____

_____

What further data did/should you collect?

_____

_____

_____

_____

What will you do with that data?

_____

_____

_____

_____

_____

How will you use that additional data to make a decision about the original assessment data?

_____

_____

_____

_____

_____

What parameters will you apply about the data under consideration that will call you to action?

_____

_____

_____

_____

_____

What decisions did you make and why?

_____

_____

_____

_____

After you answer the above questions, answer the following questions.

What is the basis for your decisions?

_____

_____

_____

_____

What will you do next and why?

_____

_____

_____

_____

What thinking skills did you use? Use the following table to explain how you used each thinking skill.

Critical Thinking Skill/Strategy	Discuss which thinking skills were used and how each was used
NOTICING Identifying Signs and Symptoms Assessing Systematically and Comprehensively Gathering Accurate Data Predicting Potential Complications	
INTERPRETING Clustering Related Information Recognizing Inconsistencies Determining Important Information to Collect Distinguishing Relevant from Irrelevant Information Judging How Much Ambiguity is Acceptable Comparing and Contrasting Managing Potential Complications Identifying Assumptions Setting Priorities Collaborating with Other Healthcare Team Members	
RESPONDING Delegating Communicating Teaching Others	
REFLECTING Evaluating Data Evaluating and Correcting Thinking	

Comparing and Contrasting Three Patients with the Same Medical Diagnosis

Activity/Tool

Select three patients with the same medical diagnosis (for example, same surgical procedure, same medical condition, same healthcare issue such as dementia, etc).

_____ Patient Information

Collect the following information on all three patients.

History:

_____

_____

_____

Current medical diagnosis:

_____

_____

_____

Other pre-existing
conditions:

_____

_____

_____

Diet:

_____

_____

Medications: _____

_____

_____

Treatments: _____

_____

_____

Limitations in function: _____

_____

_____

Procedure(s) performed: _____

_____

_____

Other pertinent information: _____

_____

_____

_____

_____

Visit each patient and perform an assessment. Complete the following table for each patient. Be sure to discuss the patient information and note reasons why diet, meds, treatments, etc., vary among the three patients.

PATIENT #1: Data Collected	How the Data are the same/different from the other patients
History	
Current Medical Diagnosis	
Other Pre-Existing Conditions	
Diet	
Medications	
Treatment	
Limitations in Function	
Procedures Performed	
Other Patient Information	

PATIENT #2: Data Collected	How the Data are the same/different from the other patients
History	
Current Medical Diagnosis	
Other Pre-Existing Conditions	
Diet	
Medications	
Treatment	
Limitations in Function	
Procedures Performed	
Other Patient Information	

PATIENT #3: Data Collected	How the Data are the same/different from the other patients
History	
Current Medical Diagnosis	
Other Pre-Existing Conditions	
Diet	
Medications	
Treatment	
Limitations in Function	
Procedures Performed	
Other Patient Information	

Review all the data for each patient and note when specific findings would be out of range and what actions to take. Note possible complications for each patient and nursing interventions to prevent those complications.

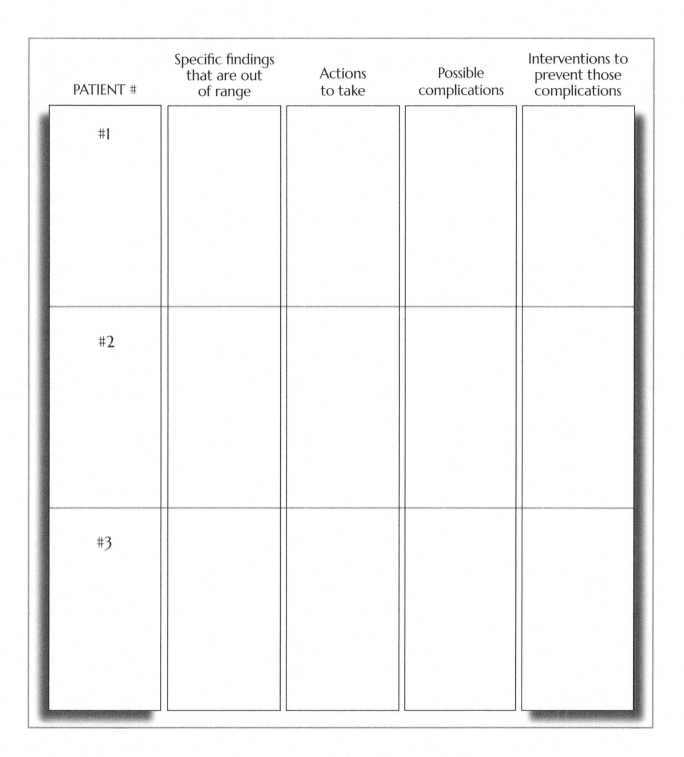

PATIENT #	Specific findings that are out of range	Actions to take	Possible complications	Interventions to prevent those complications
#1				
#2				
#3				

In addition to comparing and contrasting, what thinking skills did you use? Use the following table to explain how you used each thinking skill.

Critical Thinking Skill/Strategy	Discuss which thinking skills were used and how each was used
NOTICING Identifying Signs and Symptoms Assessing Systematically and Comprehensively Gathering Accurate Data Predicting Potential Complications	
INTERPRETING Clustering Related Information Recognizing Inconsistencies Determining Important Information to Collect Distinguishing Relevant from Irrelevant Information Judging How Much Ambiguity is Acceptable Comparing and Contrasting Managing Potential Complications Identifying Assumptions Setting Priorities Collaborating with Other Healthcare Team Members	
RESPONDING Delegating Communicating Teaching Others	
REFLECTING Evaluating Data Evaluating and Correcting Thinking	

Setting Priorities

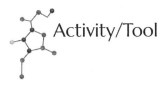Activity/Tool

After assessing your patient, list the needs the patient has at this time and categorize the identified patient needs using the following criteria in the space below. Explain your rationale.

1. First order priority need—immediate threat to health, safety, or survival

2. Second order priority need—actual problem for which immediate help has been requested by the patient or family

3. Third order priority need—actual or potential issue about which the patient or family is not aware

4. Fourth order priority need—actual or potential issue that is anticipated in the future and for which help will be needed

First Order Priority Needs with Rationale

_____

_____

_____

_____

_____

_____

_____

Second Order Priority Needs with Rationale

_____

_____

_____

_____

_____

Third Order Priority Needs with Rationale

_____

_____

_____

_____

_____

Fourth Order Priority Needs with Rationale

_____

_____

_____

_____

_____

In addition to setting priorities, what thinking skills did you use? Use the following table to explain how you used each thinking skill.

Critical Thinking Skill/Strategy	Discuss which thinking skills were used and how each was used
NOTICING Identifying Signs and Symptoms Assessing Systematically and Comprehensively Gathering Accurate Data Predicting Potential Complications	
INTERPRETING Clustering Related Information Recognizing Inconsistencies Determining Important Information to Collect Distinguishing Relevant from Irrelevant Information Judging How Much Ambiguity is Acceptable Comparing and Contrasting Managing Potential Complications Identifying Assumptions Setting Priorities Collaborating with Other Healthcare Team Members	
RESPONDING Delegating Communicating Teaching Others	
REFLECTING Evaluating Data Evaluating and Correcting Thinking	

Teaching Others

This activity focuses on discharge teaching.

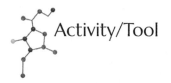Activity/Tool

Consider all the information you collected about your patient. Complete the following table.

Important information to include in discharge teaching	Why this information is important	How you obtained the information	What you will teach about this information	Method(s) used to teach the information

Once your teaching is complete, evaluate your teaching.

1. Did the patient understand what you were teaching? Explain how you know, what is the evidence?

    _____

    _____

    _____

    _____

    _____

    _____

    _____

    _____

2. Was the patient able to demonstrate that learning occurred? How do you know?

    _____

    _____

    _____

    _____

    _____

    _____

    _____

    _____

3. Is there a need to work at a later time with the patient to reinforce what was taught? Explain.

In addition to teaching others, what thinking skills did you use? Use the following table to explain how you used each thinking skill.

Critical Thinking Skill/Strategy	Discuss which thinking skills were used and how each was used
NOTICING Identifying Signs and Symptoms Assessing Systematically and Comprehensively Gathering Accurate Data Predicting Potential Complications	
INTERPRETING Clustering Related Information Recognizing Inconsistencies Determining Important Information to Collect Distinguishing Relevant from Irrelevant Information Judging How Much Ambiguity is Acceptable Comparing and Contrasting Managing Potential Complications Identifying Assumptions Setting Priorities Collaborating with Other Healthcare Team Members	
RESPONDING Delegating Communicating Teaching Others	
REFLECTING Evaluating Data Evaluating and Correcting Thinking	

Evaluating Data

Activity/Tool

Throughout the day answer the following questions.

What evaluation data will you (did you) collect for each intervention planned?

_____

_____

_____

_____

_____

_____

_____

What changes to patient care will you (did you) make based on the evaluation data?

_____

_____

_____

_____

_____

_____

_____

What findings will trigger you to take immediate action? Explain why and what actions you will take.

_____

_____

_____

_____

_____

_____

_____

_____

In addition to evaluating data, what thinking skills did you use? Use the following table to explain how you used each thinking skill.

Critical Thinking Skill/Strategy	Discuss which thinking skills were used and how each was used
NOTICING Identifying Signs and Symptoms Assessing Systematically and Comprehensively Gathering Accurate Data Predicting Potential Complications	
INTERPRETING Clustering Related Information Recognizing Inconsistencies Determining Important Information to Collect Distinguishing Relevant from Irrelevant Information Judging How Much Ambiguity is Acceptable Comparing and Contrasting Managing Potential Complications Identifying Assumptions Setting Priorities Collaborating with Other Healthcare Team Members	
RESPONDING Delegating Communicating Teaching Others	
REFLECTING Evaluating Data Evaluating and Correcting Thinking	

Evaluating and Correcting Thinking

Activity/Tool

Consider the care you provided today.

Describe one patient issue you identified. Explain what you did about that issue.

_____

_____

_____

_____

_____

_____

_____

What was the outcome and is it what you expected? Explain.

_____

_____

_____

_____

_____

_____

_____

If the expected outcome was not achieved, what will you do differently?

_____

_____

_____

_____

_____

How did your thinking impact others? Explain.

_____

_____

_____

_____

_____

Was the impact positive or negative? Explain.

_____

_____

_____

_____

_____

In addition to evaluating and correcting thinking, what thinking skills did you use? Use the following table to explain how you used each thinking skill.

Critical Thinking Skill/Strategy	Discuss which thinking skills were used and how each was used
NOTICING Identifying Signs and Symptoms Assessing Systematically and Comprehensively Gathering Accurate Data Predicting Potential Complications	
INTERPRETING Clustering Related Information Recognizing Inconsistencies Determining Important Information to Collect Distinguishing Relevant from Irrelevant Information Judging How Much Ambiguity is Acceptable Comparing and Contrasting Managing Potential Complications Identifying Assumptions Setting Priorities Collaborating with Other Healthcare Team Members	
RESPONDING Delegating Communicating Teaching Others	
REFLECTING Evaluating Data Evaluating and Correcting Thinking	

Safety and Medication Administration

This activity addresses safe administration of medications.

Activity/Tool

_____ Patient Medication

Gather information about the patient.

Medication to be administered:

_____

Classification:

_____

Patient medical diagnosis:

_____

Allergies:

_____

Surgical procedure:

_____

Chronic conditions:

_____

_____

Consider information about the medication and how it relates to the patient.

Reason why the medication is prescribed for this patient:

_____

_____

How does this medication relate to the patient's history and physical?

_____

_____

Other prescribed medications that affect the administration of this medication:

_____

_____

Expected therapeutic effects:

_____

_____

Side effects to consider:

_____

_____

When was the last time this medication was given?

_____

What were the effects of the medication the last time it was given?

_____

_____

Determine how to safely administer the medication.

Pertinent assessments
to make:

_____

_____

_____

Parameters to consider:

_____

_____

_____

Contradictions to
administering this
medication:

_____

_____

_____

Reasons to hold
(not administer)
this medication:

_____

_____

_____

Dosage that will be
administered:

_____

Route that will be used:

_____

_____

IV medication: (yes/no)

_____

Compatible with IV solution?
(yes/no)

_____

IV and medication:
explain about compatibility
between the two.

_____

_____

_____

_____

Compatible with other
meds in the line? (yes/no)

_____

Flush needed? (yes/no)

_____

IV medications:
explain about compatibility
between this medication
and others being administered.

_____

_____

_____

_____

Oral medication?

_____

Can it be crushed?

_____

Given with food?

_____

Can it be given with other medications? Explain.

_____

_____

_____

Evaluation data to collect:

_____

_____

_____

_____

When to collect evaluation data?

_____

_____

Pertinent information to document:

_____

_____

_____

_____

What thinking skills did you use? Use the following table to explain how you used each thinking skill.

Critical Thinking Skill/Strategy	Discuss which thinking skills were used and how each was used
NOTICING Identifying Signs and Symptoms Assessing Systematically and Comprehensively Gathering Accurate Data Predicting Potential Complications	
INTERPRETING Clustering Related Information Recognizing Inconsistencies Determining Important Information to Collect Distinguishing Relevant from Irrelevant Information Judging How Much Ambiguity is Acceptable Comparing and Contrasting Managing Potential Complications Identifying Assumptions Setting Priorities Collaborating with Other Healthcare Team Members	
RESPONDING Delegating Communicating Teaching Others	
REFLECTING Evaluating Data Evaluating and Correcting Thinking	

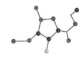

Delegating and Prioritizing Exercise

Today you have the following team members working with you: an LPN/LVN and a certified nursing assistant (CNA).

Activity/Tool

_____ Patient Information

Collect the following information on three patients.

Medical diagnosis: _____

Nursing care for today:

Activity level and assistance
needed with activity: _____

_____

Diet and assistance
needed or special needs
related to diet: _____

_____

Pain rating: _____

Medications ordered
for pain: _____

_____

Side effects of analgesics: _____

Safety issues:

_____

_____

IV fluids:

_____

_____

State of fluid balance:
(Include assessments you made to determine fluid balance.)

_____

_____

_____

Labs scheduled for today and how the labs relate to nursing care:

_____

_____

_____

Diagnostics studies scheduled for today and how the studies relate to nursing care:

_____

_____

Any dressing changes?

_____

Any suctioning?

_____

Other treatments:

_____

_____

Complete the following for each medication ordered for this patient.

Classification of the medication:

_____

Reasons why the medication was ordered:

_____

_____

_____

When it will be administered:

_____

_____

Patient teaching relative to the medication:

_____

_____

Any special instructions regarding administration of this medication:

_____

_____

Which medication for each patient is most important to administer on time and why?

_____

_____

What might happen if the medication is not administered on time?

_____

_____

_____

Visit each patient and perform a two-minute assessment of both the patient and the patient's environment. Answer the following questions based on all the information you collected.

Prioritize which patient you should care for first, second, and third. Explain.

_____

_____

_____

_____

What are the primary assessments that should be completed first for each patient? Explain.

_____

_____

_____

What nursing interventions need to be carried out for each patient?

_____

_____

_____

What interventions will you do first? Explain.

_____

_____

_____

Which of the above interventions can be delegated and to whom? Explain.

_____

_____

_____

_____

What information will be given to the person to whom the task is delegated and what information will be collected after the task is complete?

_____

_____

_____

_____

In addition to delegating and setting priorities, what thinking skills did you use? Use the following table to explain how you used each thinking skill.

Critical Thinking Skill/Strategy	Discuss which thinking skills were used and how each was used
NOTICING Identifying Signs and Symptoms Assessing Systematically and Comprehensively Gathering Accurate Data Predicting Potential Complications	
INTERPRETING Clustering Related Information Recognizing Inconsistencies Determining Important Information to Collect Distinguishing Relevant from Irrelevant Information Judging How Much Ambiguity is Acceptable Comparing and Contrasting Managing Potential Complications Identifying Assumptions Setting Priorities Collaborating with Other Healthcare Team Members	
RESPONDING Delegating Communicating Teaching Others	
REFLECTING Evaluating Data Evaluating and Correcting Thinking	

Calling the Physician/Primary Healthcare Provider (PHCP)

Activity/Tool

1. What led you to believe you need to call the physician/PHCP? Explain.

    _____

    _____

    _____

    _____

2. Have you formulated a clear picture of the problem? What is it?

    _____

    _____

    _____

    _____

3. Have you read the most recent MD/PHCP progress notes and notes from the nurse on the previous shift? What information is pertinent to this situation? Explain.

    _____

    _____

    _____

    _____

4. Should you discuss the issue with the charge nurse before calling? Why or why not?

_____

_____

_____

_____

5. What do you expect to happen as a result of this call? Explain.

_____

_____

_____

_____

6. What information do you need to collect before you call the physician/PHCP?

_____

_____

_____

_____

7. When calling, remember to:

   a. Identify self, unit, patient, room #

   b. Know the admitting diagnosis and date of admission

   c. Complete the SBAR form

S: SITUATION: Include basic demographics about your patient; name, ethnicity, age, gender, and pertinent information about the patient's condition/situation. Include patient preferences.	
B: BACKGROUND: Patient's admitting diagnosis, hospital day, medical history that might complicate the current admission, any data about what has led up to any problems the patient is currently experiencing.	
A: ASSESSMENT: Signs and symptoms that are related to the diagnosis, including vital signs, O_2 Sats, and any other pertinent assessment data.	
R: RECOMMENDATIONS: Include what you have done and the patient's response.	

What will you need to document after the call?

_____

_____

_____

_____

_____

_____

_____

_____

What thinking skills did you use? Use the following table to explain how you used each thinking skill.

Critical Thinking Skill/Strategy	Discuss which thinking skills were used and how each was used
NOTICING Identifying Signs and Symptoms Assessing Systematically and Comprehensively Gathering Accurate Data Predicting Potential Complications	
INTERPRETING Clustering Related Information Recognizing Inconsistencies Determining Important Information to Collect Distinguishing Relevant from Irrelevant Information Judging How Much Ambiguity is Acceptable Comparing and Contrasting Managing Potential Complications Identifying Assumptions Setting Priorities Collaborating with Other Healthcare Team Members	
RESPONDING Delegating Communicating Teaching Others	
REFLECTING Evaluating Data Evaluating and Correcting Thinking	

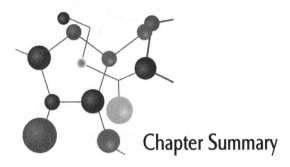

Chapter Summary

Chapter 6 activities expanded on your thinking by applying many thinking skills to one activity. These activities helped you develop skills with metacognition by requesting you to identify the thinking skills you used and how you used them. This practice with metacognition helps you develop an awareness and understanding of your own thought processes.

The majority of the activities in Chapters 5 and 6 focused on providing patient care. The nurse is also responsible for ensuring a safe healthcare environment that promotes and supports patient safety leading to improved patient outcomes. Chapter 7 provides activities that focus on (1) thinking applied to the healthcare setting, and (2) care in the community.

CHAPTER 7

Clinical Judgment/Clinical Reasoning: Applied to the Healthcare Setting and Care in the Community

As mentioned throughout this book, clinical judgment/clinical reasoning is applied to two major aspects of nursing practice. The first is engaging in direct patient care. The second is dealing with issues and problems in the healthcare setting. This chapter provides activities that directly address this second aspect of nursing. The nurse must be acutely aware of issues that arise in the healthcare setting and be prepared to deal with those issues to improve the quality of care and the quality of the healthcare system. This is a major focus known as quality improvement. As noted earlier, nurses not only engage in nursing but they also improve nursing. Improving the healthcare setting is a major factor in improving nursing. Again, the overall goal is to improve patient outcomes.

This chapter also includes a few activities that address the care of the patient in the community. Most nursing students and many nurses begin their career in the acute care setting. However, patient care is provided in a variety of settings including in the community. The community itself can be considered a "patient". The community as patient is the focus of public health nursing. The nurse must be able to use clinical judgment/clinical reasoning in any setting; therefore, this chapter also includes additional thinking activities applied to non-acute settings.

This chapter ends with overall questions for each step of the Clinical Judgment Model. This list can be applied to any situation in which the nurse applies thinking. Use this list as you analyze and evaluate your thinking. Once you have completed all the lessons in this book, keep this list handy to use as a guide as you reflect on your thinking.

Medication Administration from a Systems Perspective

"Shadow" a nurse watching and noting **every** step of the system in which medications are administered—from the time the medication prescription is written until the effects of that medication have been evaluated.

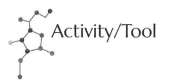

Activity/Tool

Note important aspects of the process.

_____

_____

_____

_____

Develop a description of the system used in the healthcare agency.

_____

_____

_____

_____

Identify the top five errors related to medication administration in this system.

_____

_____

_____

_____

Consider the following questions.

What is the overall process; that is, the system for safe administration of medications?

_____

_____

_____

_____

How does it work—what are the steps from prescribing to evaluating the effects of the medication?

_____

_____

_____

_____

What steps along the way lend to errors?

_____

_____

_____

_____

How can the nurse prevent errors?

_____

_____

_____

Were errors made?

_____

_____

_____

_____

What happens when an error is made?

_____

_____

_____

_____

Go to ismp.org. Identify three areas of this website that can be used to enhance safety when administering medications.

_____

_____

_____

_____

What thinking skills did you use? Use the following table to explain how you used each thinking skill.

Critical Thinking Skill/Strategy	Discuss which thinking skills were used and how each was used
NOTICING Identifying Signs and Symptoms Assessing Systematically and Comprehensively Gathering Accurate Data Predicting Potential Complications	
INTERPRETING Clustering Related Information Recognizing Inconsistencies Determining Important Information to Collect Distinguishing Relevant from Irrelevant Information Judging How Much Ambiguity is Acceptable Comparing and Contrasting Managing Potential Complications Identifying Assumptions Setting Priorities Collaborating with Other Healthcare Team Members	
RESPONDING Delegating Communicating Teaching Others	
REFLECTING Evaluating Data Evaluating and Correcting Thinking	

Implementing Safety Policies

This activity analyzes the safety policies on a nursing care unit and how they are being implemented. Visit a hospital patient care unit.

Activity/Tool

Review the unit policies related to safety. Examples might be restraints, fall risk, infection control, etc. Select three policies related to patient safety. Identify three major themes for each policy.

Policy Related to Patient Safety	Major Themes of that Policy
	1
	2
	3
	1
	2
	3
	1
	2
	3

Give at least three examples of nursing staff implementing each of these policies that you observed.

Policy #1:

_____

_____

_____

_____

_____

Policy #2:

_____

_____

_____

_____

_____

Policy #3:

_____

_____

_____

_____

_____

Give at least three examples of nursing staff *NOT IMPLEMENTING* each of these policies that you observed.

Policy #1:

_____

_____

_____

_____

_____

Policy #2:

_____

_____

_____

_____

_____

Policy #3:

_____

_____

_____

_____

_____

Explain why some of the policies were not being implemented as written.

_____

_____

_____

_____

_____

_____

_____

_____

What issues or problems may result from not adhering to each of these three policies?

_____

_____

_____

_____

_____

_____

_____

_____

What thinking skills did you use? Use the following table to explain how you used each thinking skill.

Critical Thinking Skill/Strategy	Discuss which thinking skills were used and how each was used
NOTICING Identifying Signs and Symptoms Assessing Systematically and Comprehensively Gathering Accurate Data Predicting Potential Complications	
INTERPRETING Clustering Related Information Recognizing Inconsistencies Determining Important Information to Collect Distinguishing Relevant from Irrelevant Information Judging How Much Ambiguity is Acceptable Comparing and Contrasting Managing Potential Complications Identifying Assumptions Setting Priorities Collaborating with Other Healthcare Team Members	
RESPONDING Delegating Communicating Teaching Others	
REFLECTING Evaluating Data Evaluating and Correcting Thinking	

Analyzing the Clinical Microsystem

Activity/Tool

Visit the website www.clinicalmicrosystem.org. Click on the Knowledge Center tab, then on the Workbooks tab. Under the heading Greenbooks click on Inpatient and download that workbook. Analyze a clinical unit using the following:

- Inpatient Unit Profile (page 6)

- Inpatient Unit Unplanned Activity Tracking Card (page 16)

Answer these questions.

1. What did you learn about an inpatient unit that you were not aware of?

    _____

    _____

    _____

    _____

    _____

2. What aspects of the clinical microsystem did you recognize that might lead to nurses making errors?

    _____

    _____

    _____

    _____

    _____

3. What changes can be made on the unit to prevent errors?

_____

_____

_____

_____

_____

Now download the Outpatient Primary Care workbook. Conduct the same analysis in that setting.

What are the similarities?

_____

_____

_____

_____

_____

What are the differences?

_____

_____

_____

_____

_____

List at least 3 precautions will you take in the Outpatient Primary Care setting to ensure patient safety based on the information you collected.

_____

_____

_____

_____

_____

_____

_____

_____

What thinking skills did you use? Use the following table to explain how you used each thinking skill.

Critical Thinking Skill/Strategy	Discuss which thinking skills were used and how each was used
NOTICING Identifying Signs and Symptoms Assessing Systematically and Comprehensively Gathering Accurate Data Predicting Potential Complications	
INTERPRETING Clustering Related Information Recognizing Inconsistencies Determining Important Information to Collect Distinguishing Relevant from Irrelevant Information Judging How Much Ambiguity is Acceptable Comparing and Contrasting Managing Potential Complications Identifying Assumptions Setting Priorities Collaborating with Other Healthcare Team Members	
RESPONDING Delegating Communicating Teaching Others	
REFLECTING Evaluating Data Evaluating and Correcting Thinking	

Nursing-Sensitive Indicators/Quality Improvement Measures

Activity/Tool

Visit a patient care unit in a hospital. Review their policies and procedures related to patient safety based on nursing sensitive indicators. Answer the following questions.

What nursing sensitive indicators and quality improvement projects are in use on the hospital unit?

_____

_____

_____

_____

How are the nursing sensitive quality indicators measured?

_____

_____

_____

_____

What screening tools are used?

_____

_____

_____

_____

How will you apply the nursing sensitive indicators and quality improvement processes to improve patient care?

_____

_____

_____

_____

_____

Compare the nursing-sensitive indicators used on the unit in the hospital setting above with those used in a home health setting.

Nursing Sensitive Indicators in the Hospital Setting	Nursing Sensitive Indicators in a Home Health Setting

Add more rows as needed

How are they the same?

_____

_____

_____

_____

_____

How are they different?

_____

_____

_____

_____

_____

What precautions will you take in the home health setting to ensure patient safety based on this information?

_____

_____

_____

_____

_____

What thinking skills did you use? Use the following table to explain how you used each thinking skill.

Critical Thinking Skill/Strategy	Discuss which thinking skills were used and how each was used
NOTICING Identifying Signs and Symptoms Assessing Systematically and Comprehensively Gathering Accurate Data Predicting Potential Complications	
INTERPRETING Clustering Related Information Recognizing Inconsistencies Determining Important Information to Collect Distinguishing Relevant from Irrelevant Information Judging How Much Ambiguity is Acceptable Comparing and Contrasting Managing Potential Complications Identifying Assumptions Setting Priorities Collaborating with Other Healthcare Team Members	
RESPONDING Delegating Communicating Teaching Others	
REFLECTING Evaluating Data Evaluating and Correcting Thinking	

National Patient Safety Goals Applied to a Community Setting

In an earlier chapter, you used an activity that addressed the Joint Commission's National Patient Safety Goals (NPSGs) that relate to the clinical area. Review those NPSGs. For each NPSG, discuss how you might apply those same principles to caring for a patient in a community setting.

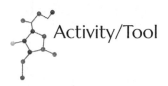 Activity/Tool

Identify the type of setting then answer the following questions.

1. What precautions should the nurse take relative to each safety goal for the patient in the community setting you selected?

    _____

    _____

    _____

    _____

    _____

    _____

2. Is there a safety goal that is the most important for patients in the community setting you selected?

    _____

    _____

    _____

    _____

    _____

    _____

3. What information about these patients is most important to communicate to other healthcare providers?

_____

_____

_____

_____

_____

_____

4. What factors about the environment indicate these safety goals are being met?

_____

_____

_____

_____

_____

_____

5. What factors about the environment indicate a need for change so the safety goals can be met?

_____

_____

_____

_____

_____

_____

Compare and contrast the implementation of the NPSGs on an inpatient unit with the implementation of the NPSGs in a community setting.

_____

_____

_____

_____

_____

_____

_____

What thinking skills did you use? Use the following table to explain how you used each thinking skill.

Critical Thinking Skill/Strategy	Discuss which thinking skills were used and how each was used
NOTICING Identifying Signs and Symptoms Assessing Systematically and Comprehensively Gathering Accurate Data Predicting Potential Complications	
INTERPRETING Clustering Related Information Recognizing Inconsistencies Determining Important Information to Collect Distinguishing Relevant from Irrelevant Information Judging How Much Ambiguity is Acceptable Comparing and Contrasting Managing Potential Complications Identifying Assumptions Setting Priorities Collaborating with Other Healthcare Team Members	
RESPONDING Delegating Communicating Teaching Others	
REFLECTING Evaluating Data Evaluating and Correcting Thinking	

Conflict Resolution

Conflicts are inevitable. You cannot avoid conflicts in the healthcare setting. Therefore, the nurse must be skilled at resolving conflict. This activity focuses on an awareness of conflict resolution in the healthcare setting.

Activity/Tool

Identify a conflict in the healthcare setting. Describe the conflict, the nature of the issue, and who is involved.

_____

_____

_____

_____

_____

_____

Plan ways to handle the conflict you identified.

_____

_____

_____

_____

_____

_____

_____

_____

What interactions of the healthcare professionals contributed to the conflict?

_____

_____

_____

_____

_____

_____

How was the conflict actually handled?

_____

_____

_____

_____

_____

_____

Compare the way you planned to handle the conflict with the way the conflict was actually handled.

_____

_____

_____

_____

_____

_____

Which approach to handling the conflict was better—the way you planned or the way the conflict was actually handled? Explain.

_____

_____

_____

_____

_____

_____

_____

_____

What thinking skills did you use? Use the following table to explain how you used each thinking skill.

Critical Thinking Skill/Strategy	Discuss which thinking skills were used and how each was used
NOTICING Identifying Signs and Symptoms Assessing Systematically and Comprehensively Gathering Accurate Data Predicting Potential Complications	
INTERPRETING Clustering Related Information Recognizing Inconsistencies Determining Important Information to Collect Distinguishing Relevant from Irrelevant Information Judging How Much Ambiguity is Acceptable Comparing and Contrasting Managing Potential Complications Identifying Assumptions Setting Priorities Collaborating with Other Healthcare Team Members	
RESPONDING Delegating Communicating Teaching Others	
REFLECTING Evaluating Data Evaluating and Correcting Thinking	

Analyzing the Electronic Medical Record

Information technology is a major focus in today's healthcare setting. The electronic medical record is convenient to use. Many aspects of these systems were implemented to ensure safe patient care. The nurse must determine if the systems are properly implemented to ensure safety, if there are breakdowns, or if nurses are using "work arounds" to save time. Work arounds are short cuts that bypass some of the safety features that are deemed time consuming. These work arounds often negate the safety aspects of these systems.

Activity/Tool

Examine an electronic medical record system in a healthcare setting. Answer the following questions.

1.   Describe the computer information system on the unit. How does its use contribute to safe nursing care?

_____

_____

_____

_____

_____

_____

_____

_____

_____

2. Discuss how missing data on the admission database and inconsistencies in documentation affect the accuracy of the information being used to make clinical decisions in the healthcare setting. Was there any information missing in the electronic record and how did that affect safe nursing practice?

_____

_____

_____

_____

_____

_____

_____

_____

3. Discuss the benefits of having access to advanced technology in the healthcare setting, such as an electronic medical record and computerized order entry. Note specific advantages of the system you are analyzing.

_____

_____

_____

_____

_____

_____

_____

_____

4. What is the nurse's obligation and accountability for ensuring proper documentation of clinical data to support coordination of care?

_____

_____

_____

_____

_____

_____

_____

_____

What thinking skills did you use? Use the following table to explain how you used each thinking skill.

Critical Thinking Skill/Strategy	Discuss which thinking skills were used and how each was used
NOTICING Identifying Signs and Symptoms Assessing Systematically and Comprehensively Gathering Accurate Data Predicting Potential Complications	
INTERPRETING Clustering Related Information Recognizing Inconsistencies Determining Important Information to Collect Distinguishing Relevant from Irrelevant Information Judging How Much Ambiguity is Acceptable Comparing and Contrasting Managing Potential Complications Identifying Assumptions Setting Priorities Collaborating with Other Healthcare Team Members	
RESPONDING Delegating Communicating Teaching Others	
REFLECTING Evaluating Data Evaluating and Correcting Thinking	

Windshield Survey

Just as you assess a patient, you assess a community. This tool guides you through a community assessment. Many thinking skills are used in the collection of this data and the analysis of the data to determine community needs.

Activity/Tool

BOUNDARIES

Are there geographic or physical boundaries such as a highway, railroad, lake, river, a different terrain, presence of industrial or commercial units along with residential?

_____

_____

_____

_____

Does the neighborhood have an identity, a name? If so, is it displayed?

_____

_____

_____

_____

Are there unofficial names?

_____

_____

_____

_____

Are there sub-communities within the area?

_____

_____

_____

_____

HOUSING AND ZONING

How old are the houses? What is the style of houses and what types of materials were used in their construction?

_____

_____

_____

_____

Are all the neighborhood houses similar?

_____

_____

_____

_____

If not, how would you characterize the differences?

_____

_____

_____

_____

Are there single or multi-family homes or both?

_____

_____

_____

_____

What size are the lots (approximately)?

_____

_____

_____

_____

Are there signs of disrepair such as broken doors, steps, windows, and un-
kempt yards?

_____

_____

_____

_____

Are there vacant houses?

_____

_____

_____

_____

Does the neighborhood show signs of improvements or signs of decay?

_____

_____

_____

_____

Is it "alive"? How would you decide?

_____

_____

_____

_____

Is there trash, abandoned cars, boarded up buildings, rubble, dilapidated buildings, and cluttered vacant lots?

_____

_____

_____

_____

Is there evidence of poor drainage, potential disease, and breeding places for disease producing organisms to grow?

_____

_____

_____

_____

PARKS AND RECREATIONAL AREAS

Are there parks and recreational areas in the neighborhood? Are there green spaces?

_____

_____

_____

_____

Is the open space public or private?

_____

_____

_____

_____

Who uses these spaces?

_____

_____

_____

_____

COMMON AREAS

Are there areas where people congregate? Describe these areas.

_____

_____

_____

_____

What groups of people congregate and at what hours?

_____

_____

_____

_____

Do these gathering areas have a sense of territoriality or are they open to strangers?

_____

_____

_____

_____

STORES

What supermarkets or neighborhood stores are available?

_____

_____

_____

_____

How do residents travel to the store?

_____

_____

_____

_____

Are there drug stores, laundries, dry cleaners, and other services in the area?

_____

_____

_____

_____

TRANSPORTATION

How do people get in and out of the neighborhood?

_____

_____

_____

_____

What is the condition of the streets?

_____

_____

_____

_____

Is there a major highway near the neighborhood?

_____

_____

_____

_____

Is public transportation available and is that public transportation available to all in the area such as the elderly and disabled?

_____

_____

_____

_____

SERVICE CENTERS

Are there social agencies, recreation centers, schools, and libraries?

_____

_____

_____

_____

_____

Are there healthcare providers such as physicians, dentists, clinics, emergency departments, hospitals, and long-term care facilities?

_____

_____

_____

_____

_____

PEOPLE ON THE STREET

Who is on the streets, such as women, children, teenagers, community health nurses, collection agents, salespeople?

_____

_____

_____

_____

How are they dressed?

_____

_____

_____

_____

What animals do you see, such as strays, pets, other?

_____

_____

_____

_____

PROTECTIVE SERVICES

Is there evidence of police in the area?

_____

_____

_____

Is there evidence of fire protection in the area?

_____

_____

_____

RACE

Are there various racial groups in the neighborhood?

_____

_____

_____

How many are there?

_____

_____

_____

ETHNICITY AND RELIGION

What churches & church schools are in the neighborhood?

_____

_____

_____

How many are there?

_____

_____

CLASS

How would you categorize the residents: upper, lower, upper middle, middle, working, etc.? On what do you base this judgment?

_____

_____

_____

_____

_____

HEALTH AND SAFETY

Is there evidence of accidents, substance abuse, poor lighting on streets, poor sidewalk/street conditions? On what do you base this judgment?

_____

_____

_____

_____

_____

Are cyclists wearing helmets?

_____

Are sidewalks clear of snow/ice (in winter), obstacles?

_____

SUMMARY OF YOUR OVERALL ASSESSMENT OF THE COMMUNITY

What is your impression of this community?

_____

_____

_____

_____

Conduct an internet search of the community. What are the major health concerns for this area?

_____

_____

_____

_____

Describe the populations in the community that are the most vulnerable and at risk for not receiving health care.

_____

_____

_____

_____

_____

What thinking skills did you use? Use the following table to explain how you used each thinking skill.

Critical Thinking Skill/Strategy	Discuss which thinking skills were used and how each was used
NOTICING Identifying Signs and Symptoms Assessing Systematically and Comprehensively Gathering Accurate Data Predicting Potential Complications	
INTERPRETING Clustering Related Information Recognizing Inconsistencies Determining Important Information to Collect Distinguishing Relevant from Irrelevant Information Judging How Much Ambiguity is Acceptable Comparing and Contrasting Managing Potential Complications Identifying Assumptions Setting Priorities Collaborating with Other Healthcare Team Members	
RESPONDING Delegating Communicating Teaching Others	
REFLECTING Evaluating Data Evaluating and Correcting Thinking	

Overall Questions Related to Each Step of the Thinking Model

This chapter ends with an overall look at the steps of the Clinical Judgment Model. Following are a number of questions you can use to help guide your thinking. Consider each of these questions as you are working through a problem in any learning or practice environment.

NOTICING: WHAT DID/SHOULD YOU NOTICE?

1. What do you know about this type of situation that will influence what you should notice?

2. What issues/problems/concerns are important to this situation?

3. What information about each issue/problem/concern do you need to remember and apply to this situation?

4. Is the situation as you would expect it to be based on your past experiences with this type of situation?

5. Is there additional information you need to look up that you are not remembering that should be included in your "noticing" or that you need to be sure you are remembering correctly?

6. What does the textbook say about this situation?

7. Is there a clinical protocol, core measure, or other guide that presents concerns that require your attention for this type of situation?

8. What assessment aids should you use to be sure you "notice" everything?

9. What factors about previously collected assessment data (trending data) for this patient should you consider and include as you are assessing?

10. Are you making assumptions about this situation, patient, person, etc. that may be biased?

INTERPRETING: WHAT DOES IT MEAN?

1. Are you able to make sense of the patient situation (patient problem/issue, clinical unit problem, interprofessional issue, etc.)?

2. Did any of the assessment data trigger the identification of other data to collect to support or enhance the meaning of the collected data? Any interrelated issues/problems/concerns?

3. What factors about the patient/situation did you use to guide your interpretation of this situation?

4. Are you able to identify what information is most important in this situation?

5. Of the important information, which data are relevant to the immediate concern?

6. What "rules" are you applying to this situation and how are you applying each rule? How much "wiggle room" do you have with that rule and still be in the safe zone for this patient?

7. What findings will trigger a call to another healthcare provider? How will you determine which healthcare provider to call?

8. What data would trigger a call to the rapid response team or other emergency intervention?

9. What is the basis for how you prioritize your actions?

RESPONDING: WHAT DO YOU DO?

1. Can you delegate any intervention to other personnel?

2. Is your communication clear and effective?

3. Are your interventions within the scope of practice of your level of nursing?

4. Are your interventions within ethical and professional guidelines?

5. What teaching needs to be done and who needs the teaching?

REFLECTING: WHAT WAS THE EFFECT OF YOUR THINKING?

1. What did you expect to occur as a result of your actions and did it occur? If not, why?

2. Was there anything unexpected as a result of your actions? Are these unexpected results acceptable?

3. How did the patient, family, or staff respond to your intervention?

4. What worked?

5. What didn't work?

6. What can you do better?

7. What do you need to work on?

8. What will you do differently the next time you encounter this type of situation?

9. What can you learn from the unexpected results, and how can you use this learning in future similar situations?

10. What feedback did you receive on your actions and what will you do with that feedback?

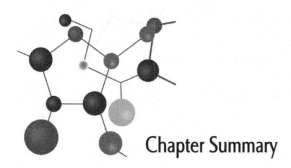

Chapter Summary

Chapter 7 provided activities that applied your clinical judgment/clinical reasoning to issues in the healthcare setting and to nursing in the community. These are just examples of the myriad of types of issues, situations, problems, and other concerns you will continuously encounter in a typical day as a nurse. Just as you constantly work to perfect all the psychomotor skills you will perform for patients, you must constantly work to improve your thinking.

The nurse's ability to engage in the thinking needed to make sound, quality clinical judgments is perhaps the number one factor affecting patient outcomes. Remember, improving patient outcomes is every nurse's goal and high-level thinking and clinical judgment/clinical reasoning help make that goal a reality.

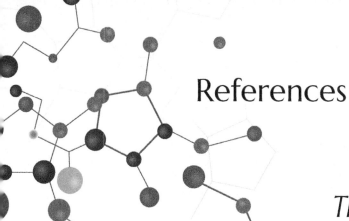

References

Think Like a Nurse: A Handbook

Ambrose, S. A., Bridges, M. W., DiPietro, M., Lovett, M. C., & Norman, M. K. (2010). *How learning works: 7 research-based principles for smart teaching*. San Francisco: John Wiley.

Benner, P. (2001). *From novice to expert: Excellence and power in clinical nursing practice*. (Commemorative Edition). Upper Saddle River, NJ: Prentice Hall.

Brown, P. C., Roediger, H. L., & McDaniel, M. A. (2014). *Make it stick: The science of successful learning*. Cambridge, MA: The Belknap Press of Harvard University Press.

Cannon, S., & Boswell, C. (Eds.) (2016). *Evidence-based teaching in nursing: A foundation for educators*, (2nd ed.), Burlington, MA: Jones & Bartlett.

Cappelletti, A., Engel, J. K., & & Prentice, D. (2014). Systematic review of clinical judgment and reasoning in nursing. *Journal of Nursing Education, 45,* 453-458.

Caputi, L. (2016). The Caputi model for teaching thinking in nursing, In L. Caputi, (Ed.), *Innovations in nursing education: Building the future of nursing,* (Vol. 3), p. 3-12. Philadelphia: Wolters Kluwer.

Caputi, L. (2010a). An introduction to developing critical thinking in nursing education. In L. Caputi, (Ed.), *Teaching nursing: The art and science*, (Vol. 2), p. 381-390. Glen Ellyn, IL: DuPage Press.

Caputi, L. (2010b). Operationalizing Critical Thinking. In L. Caputi, (Ed.), *Teaching nursing: The art and science*, (Vol. 2), p. 391-412. Glen Ellyn, IL: DuPage Press.

Erickson, H. L., & Lanning, L. A. (2014). *Transitioning to concept-based curriculum and instruction: How to bring content and process together*. Thousand Oaks, CA: Corwin.

Hines, C. B., & Wood, F. G. (2016). Clinical judgment scripts as a strategy to foster clinical judgments. *Journal of Nursing Education, 55*(12), 691-695.

Institute of Medicine (IOM). (2011). *The future of nursing: Leading change, advancing health*. Washington, DC: The National Academies Press.

Jessee, M. A., & Tanner, C. A. (2016). Pursuing improvement in clinical reasoning: Development of the clinical coaching interactions inventory. *Journal of Nursing Education, 55*(9), 495-504.

Koharchik, L., Caputi, L., Robb, M., & Culleiton, A. (2015). Fostering clinical reasoning in nursing students. *American Journal of Nursing, 115,* (1), 58-61.

Lasater, K. (2011). Clinical judgment: The last frontier for evaluation. *Nurse Education in Process, 11,* 86-92.

Levett-Jones, T., Hoffman, K., Dempsey, J., Jeong, S., Noble, D., Norton, C., Roche, J., & Hickey, N. (2009). The 'five rights' of clinical reasoning: An educational model to enhance nursing students' ability to identify and mange clinically 'at risk' patients. *Nurse Educator Today, 30*, 515-520.

Makary, M. A., & Daniel, M. (2016). Medical error—the third leading cause of death in the US. *British Medical Journal,* 353: doi: http://dx.doi.org/10.1136/bmj.i2139

McNelis, A., Ironside, P., Ebright, P., Dreifuerst, K., Zvonar, S., & Conner, S. (2014). Learning nursing practice: A multisite, multimethod investigation of clinical education. *Journal of Nursing Regulation, 4*(4), 30-35.

Nielsen, A. & Lasater, K. (2017), Clinical judgment. In. J. Giddens, Ed., *Concepts for nursing practice*, (2nd ed). St. Louis: Elsevier.

Nilson, L. B. (2013). *Creating self-regulated learners.* Sterling, VA: Stylus.

Panadero, E., Alonso-Tapia, J., & Reche, E. (2013). Rubrics vs. self-assessment scripts effect on self-regulation, performance, and self-efficacy in pre-service teachers. *Studies in Educational Evaluation, 39,* 125-132.

Paul, R., & Elder, L. (2014). *The miniature guide to critical thinking: Concepts and tools* (7th ed.). Dillon Beach, CA: The Foundation for Critical Thinking.

Purling, A., & King, L. (2012). A literature review: Graduate nurses' preparedness for recognising and responding to the deteriorating patient. *Journal of Clinical Nursing,* 21, 3451-3465.

Rubenfeld, M. G., & Scheffer, B. K. (2015). *Critical thinking TACTICS for nurses: Achieving the IOM competencies.* (3rd ed.). Sudbury, MA: Jones & Bartlett.

Tanner, C. (2006). Thinking like a nurse: A research-based model of clinical judgment in nursing. *Journal of Nursing Education, 45*(6), 204-211.

Made in the USA
Columbia, SC
28 August 2019